Nutrition for OUTDOOR RECREATION

MARISA MICHAEL, MSc, RDN, CSSD

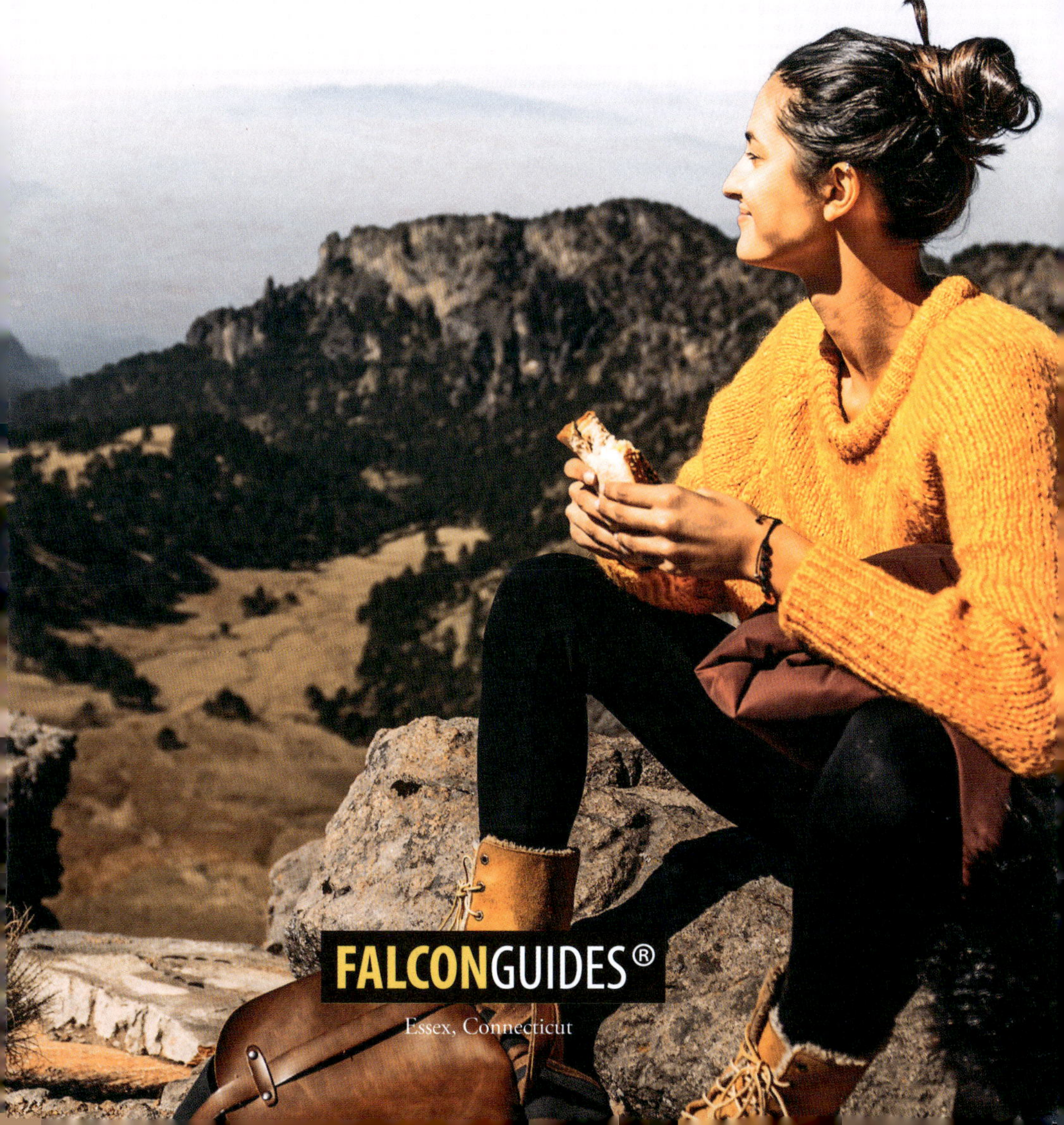

FALCONGUIDES®
Essex, Connecticut

FALCONGUIDES®

An imprint of The Globe Pequot Publishing Group, Inc.
64 South Main Street
Essex, CT 06426
www.globepequot.com

Falcon and FalconGuides are registered trademarks and Make Adventure Your Story is a trademark of The Globe Pequot Publishing Group, Inc.

Copyright © 2025 Marisa Michael
Photos by Marisa Michael unless otherwise noted

All rights reserved. No part of this book may be reproduced in any form or by any electronic or mechanical means, including information storage and retrieval systems, without written permission from the publisher, except by a reviewer who may quote passages in a review.

British Library Cataloguing in Publication Information available

Library of Congress Cataloging-in-Publication Data
Names: Michael, Marisa, author.
Title: Nutrition for outdoor recreation / Marisa Michael, MSc, RDN, CSSD.
Description: Essex, Connecticut : FalconGuides, [2025] | Includes
   bibliographical references and index.
Identifiers: LCCN 2025001073 (print) | LCCN 2025001074 (ebook) | ISBN
   9781493090693 (paper ; acid-free paper) | ISBN 9781493090709 (epub)
Subjects: LCSH: Outdoor recreation. | Nutrition. | Diet therapy. | BISAC:
   HEALTH & FITNESS / Diet & Nutrition / Macrobiotics | SPORTS & RECREATION
   / Hiking
Classification: LCC GV191.6 .M54 2025 (print) | LCC GV191.6 (ebook) | DDC
   613.2—dc23/eng/20250417
LC record available at https://lccn.loc.gov/2025001073
LC ebook record available at https://lccn.loc.gov/2025001074

Printed in India

The author and The Globe Pequot Publishing Group, Inc., assume no liability for accidents happening to, or injuries sustained by, readers who engage in the activities described in this book.

Contents

INTRODUCTION	v
Chapter 1: Nutrition Basics	**1**
General Nutrition	1
Energy	2
Macronutrients	6
Micronutrients	13
Fluids	16
The Wrap-Up	23
Chapter 2: Meal Planning, Nutrient Timing, and Nutrition Periodization	**25**
The Plate Method	26
How to Calculate Your Own Nutrient Needs	28
Meal Timing	36
Nutrition Periodization	39
The Wrap-Up	40
Chapter 3: Special Nutrition Situations	**42**
Altitude	43
Heat	48
Cold	51
Van and RV Life	53
Vegan and Vegetarian Diets	56
Troubleshooting Digestive Issues	60
Youth and Adolescent Nutrition	64
Masters Nutrition	67
Female Athletes	68
Para/Adaptive Athletes	72
Traveling Nutrition	75
Nutrition for Injury and Surgery	77
The Wrap-Up	80

Chapter 4: Supplements — 82

    Introduction — 82
    How to Select a Safe Supplement — 83
    Creatine — 85
    Beta-alanine — 86
    Sodium Bicarbonate — 87
    Caffeine — 88
    Nitrates — 90
    Fish Oil/Omega-3s — 91
    Collagen — 92
    Protein Powders — 94
    The Wrap-Up — 96

Chapter 5: Fueling Your Adventure — 99

    Snow Sports — 100
    Hiking — 104
    Trail Running — 111
    Climbing — 120
    Biking — 128
    Water Sports — 131
    Camping — 134
    The Wrap-Up — 141

Chapter 6: Disordered Eating and Relative Energy Deficiency in Sport (REDs) — 145

    Eating Disorder vs. Disordered Eating — 147
    Relative Energy Deficiency in Sport (REDs) — 154
    Disordered Eating and REDs — 157
    Overtraining and REDs — 158
    Relationship of Body Weight to Sports Performance — 158
    How to Foster a Good Relationship with Food/Body/Exercise — 160
    The Wrap-Up — 163

Chapter 7: Sample Meal Plans and Selected Recipes — 165

    Introduction — 165
    Sample Meal Plans — 166
    Recipes — 176

ACKNOWLEDGMENTS — 188
INDEX — 189
ABOUT THE AUTHOR — 193

Introduction

I am standing on the edge of the Grand Canyon. I've just arrived and am considering a short hike before the sun sets. All around me is stunning beauty . . . and posted signs depicting a man vomiting! It reads: "Hiking the Colorado River and back in one day is not recommended due to long distance, extreme heat, and a nearly 5,000-foot (1,500-m) elevation change. If you think you have the fitness and expertise to attempt this extremely strenuous hike, please seek advice from a park ranger at the Backcountry Information Center."

The message is clear: *Don't hike if you aren't prepared*. Part of that preparation includes a fueling and hydration plan to prevent emergencies or death. But how do you know if you got it right?

Outdoor recreation is all about connecting with nature, feeling the joy of being outdoors, and finding satisfaction in doing hard things. It's a true wonder to be immersed in the beauty of a forest, float effortlessly in a lake, or reach the summit of a mountain.

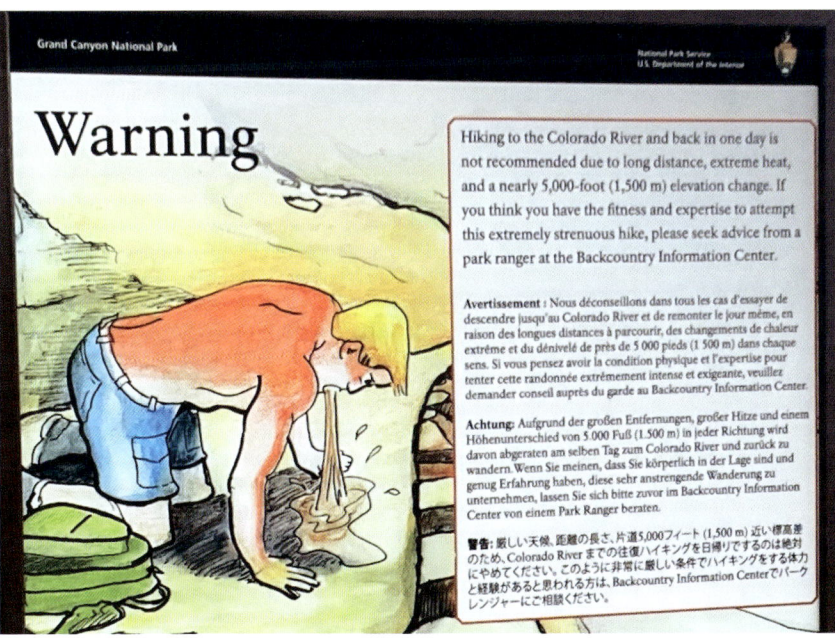

We spend a lot of time planning, packing, training, and traveling to get to these places. We also spend a lot of money! Even the budget-conscious athlete can find themself spending several hundred dollars on gear. Yet with all this planning and spending, many are missing one key thing: *nutrition*.

Fueling properly for both adventure and life can promote longevity in outdoor recreation, lower injury risk, and prevent backcountry emergencies such as heat stroke or dehydration. Beyond this, the right nutrition knowledge—implemented well—can make the difference between an amazing hike and a miserable one. If you understand how to fuel and hydrate, you will find outdoor recreation safer and more enjoyable.

That's where this book comes in! It can solve your nutrition problems, such as:

- The backpacker that needs more food at a lighter weight
- The mountain biker who keeps getting cramps
- The skier whose food keeps getting frozen
- The paddler who became dehydrated
- The climber who was told she should lose weight to send her project
- The outdoor athlete who is tired of confusing, conflicting nutrition information

This book will take you through the basics of energy systems in the body, macronutrients, micronutrients, and fluids/electrolytes to build a foundation of evidence-based nutrition knowledge. From there, it will layer in specific, practical, and actionable steps for all sorts of outdoor scenarios. You'll then be an unstoppable outdoor athlete, armed with a plan for any adventure, energized and fueled to take on the wilderness.

You got this!

~Marisa Michael

This book contains general information only and not nutrition or medical advice. Always consult with your health care professional before undergoing any diet or lifestyle change.

1
NUTRITION BASICS

GENERAL NUTRITION

Jane was competing in a 30K trail run. She thought she had her fueling and hydration dialed in. She had practiced beforehand with training runs. She tested out the products to make sure her stomach could tolerate them. She even calculated how many ounces of fluid per hour she needed to drink.

And yet, during her race, she began having serious stomach issues. Bloating and cramping made her slow down and walk. She drank more fluid, thinking she was dehydrated. But that wasn't the problem—instead, her sports drink of choice was too concentrated. Drinking more of it only exacerbated her symptoms. She was able to finish the race but felt terrible and had a disappointing finish time.

How could she have avoided this? Knowing how many grams of carbs she was taking in per hour, knowing how much and what type of carbs her stomach could tolerate, and understanding the signs of dehydration would have helped.

As the saying goes, you don't know what you don't know. As an outdoor athlete, there are many nutrition principles that you can leverage to make each adventure a success. But if you don't know them, you're missing out on huge potential.

Nutrition can be complex, but there are some general nutrition principles you can utilize in your outdoor adventures that will be the foundation for everything you do. There are a lot of nutrition myths and misinformation out there. Understanding what is true and how to apply it can optimize your adventures.

This book will guide you toward these main goals:

- Eat enough to support basic body processes.
- Eat enough to support training and movement (before, during, and after activity).
- Eat a healthful diet made of mostly whole grains, fruits/vegetables, nuts/seeds, dairy products, and lean protein.*

---

* Vegans and those with special dietary needs or preferences may have different diet patterns they need to follow. For more on vegan and vegetarian diets, see Chapter 3.

- Refuel and rehydrate after workouts to promote recovery.
- Maintain a good relationship with food, body, and sport.

This book is designed to be read cover-to-cover or as individual chapters. You may find yourself wanting to flip to certain sections that apply to you. Spend some time in this chapter and then start reading whatever interests you. Or read it cover-to-cover! Either way, you'll get the information you need. Please note that if you read it all the way through, you may find a concept or two that you've already read somewhere else. Some redundancy had to occur to make the chapters work as stand-alone pieces. Either way you choose to read it, you will find useful information.

As an athlete, you need to know nutrition basics to perform at your best, prevent injury, and optimize recovery. Understanding fueling will also help you stay safe. For instance, the rangers at the Grand Canyon have a huge concern with keeping people safe. They do not want hikers to become dehydrated or suffer from heat exhaustion.

While this section may seem basic to some, it will be the foundation for the rest of the nutrition sections in this book, so it's helpful to review it.

You'll notice that the word *fueling* will come up often in this book. Fueling refers to a specific strategy to provide energy for outdoor activities. Fueling is different than a normal everyday eating pattern. For example, a sports drink with added sugar and salt may be needed for a hot hike, but in general, it's not a healthful diet pattern to add sugar and salt to your everyday foods. While fueling does support health and performance, it has a different function than adopting a day-to-day diet pattern. Your overall diet pattern is important to health, and so is fueling properly.

ENERGY

What provides energy for your body? Food! (Did you answer caffeine? We'll get to that later in Chapter 4.) Food provides energy for the body.

Energy is measured in calories (some countries use kilojoules). A calorie is the amount of energy needed to raise 1 gram of water 1 degree Celsius. Since this is such a tiny amount, the calories we see listed on food labels are actually kilocalories, or Calories with a capital C. For simplicity in this book, I will use "calorie" to refer to kilocalories, since that is what most people commonly use.

Adequate energy from food is essential for your body to have the resources it needs to function. Your body uses this energy to maintain normal body processes, such as heart rate, breathing, producing new cells to maintain tissues, immune system regulation, digestion, and more.

Your body needs a certain amount of baseline calories to exist, and then you need additional calories to do whatever else you ask your body to do. Working, daily household tasks, exercising, and even thinking require extra calories. Getting the right amount to support your body will help you be healthy.

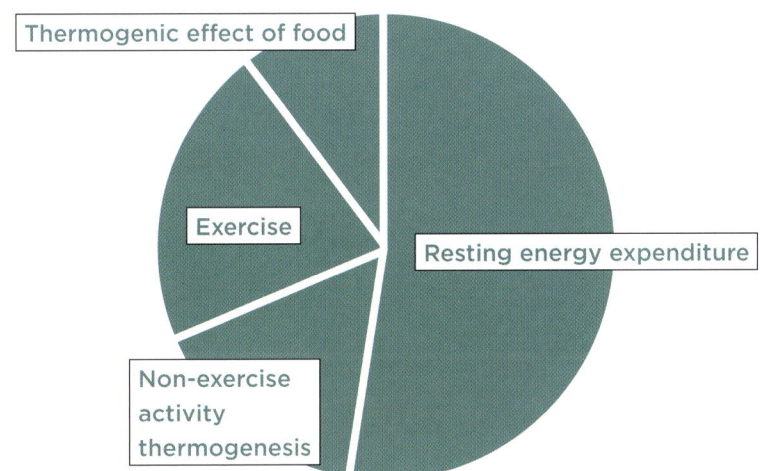

TOTAL ENERGY EXPENDITURE

Your total energy expenditure—or the amount of calories your body burns each day—is made up of:

- Resting energy expenditure (those baseline needs mentioned above)
- Intentional exercise
- Activity that isn't intentional exercise (chores, fidgeting, sitting, standing); called non-exercise activity thermogenesis, or NEAT
- Thermogenic effect of food (the energy needed to metabolize food)

1 / NUTRITION BASICS

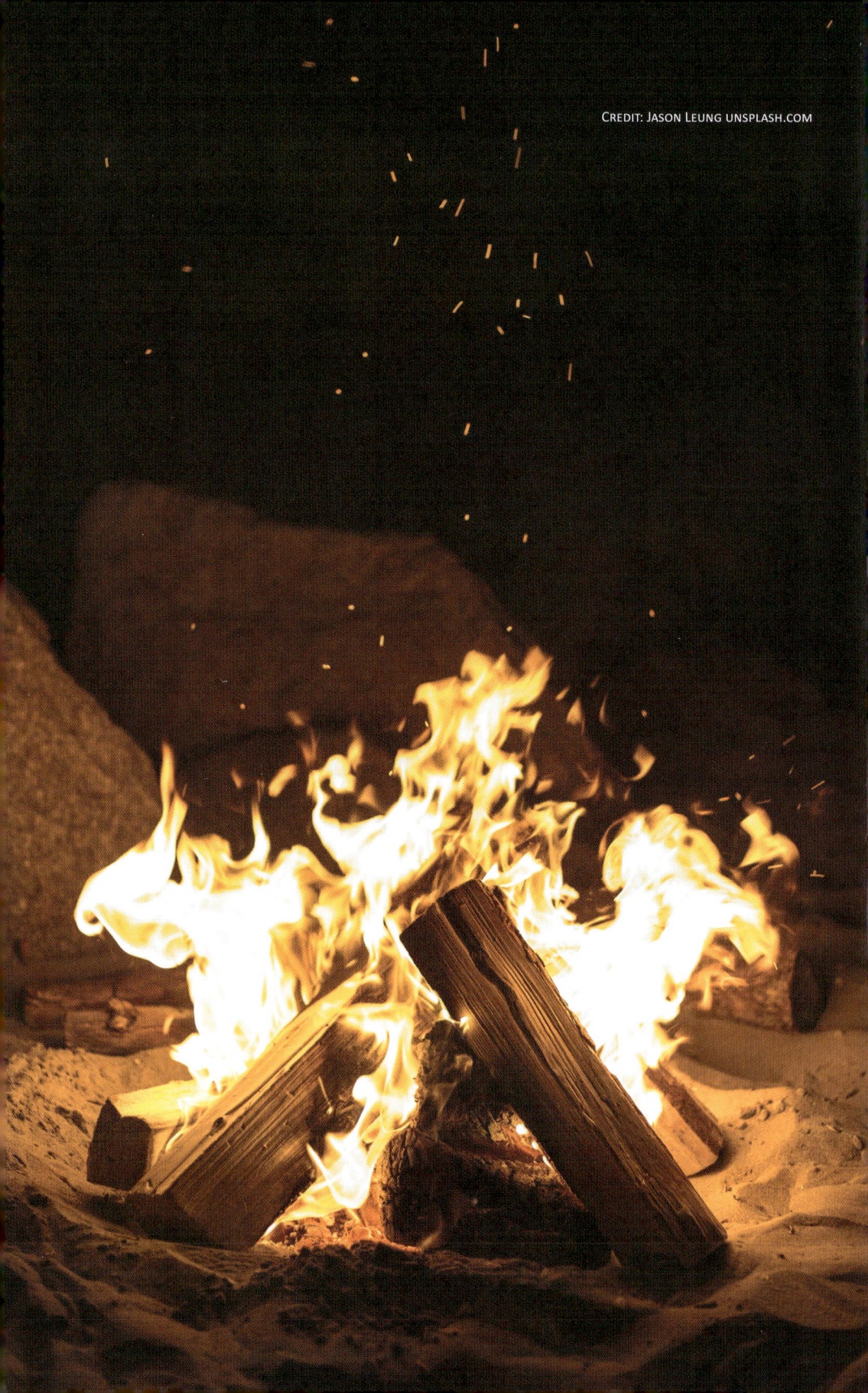
Credit: Jason Leung unsplash.com

I like the campfire analogy for energy needs. Think of it this way: A campfire needs the right amount of fuel at the right time to burn efficiently. If you add too many big logs too soon, the fire is snuffed out. Failing to provide too little fuel when the fire is burning brightly also will cause the fire to die. Putting the right size and amount of fuel in the form of tinder, sticks, and logs will help it burn hot and last a long time.

Similarly, energy needs vary from person to person based on their gender, age, body composition, and activity level. They also vary if you are stressed, injured, or sick. Energy needs also fluctuate from day to day or week to week—they aren't always exact or static.

Just like adding logs or tinder at the right time to the campfire will help it burn brightly, being aware of what type of energy your body may need (carbs, fats, or protein), in the right *amount* at the right *time* can optimize your performance and recovery.

For example, simple carbohydrate with very little fiber, like gummy bears, in general is not recommended for an overall healthy diet pattern, but gummy bears are the perfect fuel for providing quick energy during a cross-country ski day. Eating a slice of pizza before doing a series of running sprints may cause gastrointestinal troubles, but it is perfectly fine after a long day of climbing. Applying basic nutrition principles based on energy systems can help you know how to fuel for all kinds of scenarios.

ENERGY SYSTEMS

"Energy systems" refers to the processes in your body and within the cells to metabolize nutrients and create energy for movement. Understanding these energy systems and the substrates (substrates = source of energy utilized in the cell) involved will help you apply practical nutrition to any outdoor situation.

For example, if you understand that hiking at a steady state with a moderate heart rate, your body uses mostly carbohydrate and fat, you can plan to bring the right kinds of foods with you. If you know that protein contributes to muscle building and repair, you can use that information to consume more protein at the right time during your post-workout recovery window.

And, if you know that an all-out intense move—such as a dyno while bouldering or a sprint to overtake a competitor in a mountain biking race—utilizes primarily carbohydrate in your body, you will know to eat simple carbs before and during the activity.

There are three main energy systems in the human body:

Adenosine Triphosphate-Phosphocreatine System (ATP-PC System)
This is an anaerobic system. It is used for powerful, explosive movements such as a power lift or a dyno. It can only supply energy for about 10 seconds.

Anaerobic Glycolysis (also called the Lactic Acid System or the Anaerobic Energy System)
This system is used for short, intense movements such as a sprint. It supplies energy for around 10 seconds to a few minutes. This system contributes to that burning sensation in your muscles when you're doing something difficult for a short time. The main substrate used in this system is glucose, which is a simple sugar (carbohydrate).

Aerobic Metabolism (also called the Aerobic Energy System)
This is the main energy system used in most outdoor activities. It is the system your cells are using when you're doing a moderate or low-intensity activity that you can do for a long time, like hiking, paddling, or skiing. This system uses both carbohydrate and fat.

These systems are sometimes used simultaneously in the body—the cells do not shut down one abruptly at the 10-second mark and then switch to another one. The main thing to note here is that carbohydrate is a key substrate, or source of energy, for most body processes. Cells in the body, including your brain and muscles, prefer glucose as their main source of energy. Throughout this book, you'll see a lot of recommendations for using carbohydrate to fuel your adventures. That's because it is used in the body's energy systems.

MACRONUTRIENTS

Macronutrients are nutrients that provide energy. Or, in other words, nutrients that provide calories. These are carbohydrate, protein, fat, and alcohol. Let's look at each one.

CARBOHYDRATE
Role in the body: Many popular diets eliminate or limit carbohydrates (commonly called "carbs"), but carbohydrates are an important macronutrient for sports performance. Whether you are climbing, skiing, hiking, lifting weights, or anything else, your body needs carbohydrates to fuel those movements.

Carbohydrate is the fuel for the anaerobic energy system and the aerobic energy system. If you are doing a moderate-paced endurance exercise, your body is using a mix of both carbohydrate and fat to fuel that workout. If you are doing an intense move, such as a sprint or power lift, your body uses carbohydrate to fuel that movement. Carbohydrate provides 4 calories per gram.

The food you eat, including carbohydrates, also keeps your blood sugar regulated and provides fuel for your brain. Glucose is a form of simple sugar (carbohydrate) in your blood. It serves as fuel for your cells and brain. Your body likes to keep blood sugar levels regular so you can feel optimal and perform your best.

Glycogen is a storage form of glucose. It is stored in your liver and skeletal muscles. Glycogen helps keep your blood sugar stable by breaking down into glucose when you are sleeping or fasting. It also is onboard fuel in your muscles to power muscle contractions.

Most people have around 1,200–1,400 calories of glycogen in their muscles and liver. If you exercise for about 2 to 3 hours without eating any food or drinking any fluids that provide calories and carbohydrates, you can run out of fuel and "bonk." This is common in endurance events such as marathon and triathlon, as well as cross-country skiing or all-day adventures.

Bonking simply means your body runs out of fuel to power your exercise and your blood sugar drops. Symptoms include feeling weak, shaky, and lethargic, with heavy legs and fatigue. Some people also feel nauseated or irritable. You can prevent bonking by eating regularly, about 30–60 grams of quickly digestible carbohydrates per hour (such as a white bagel, gummies/chews, juice, honey, or sports drink), or even up to 90–120 grams per hour for long endurance events.

You can recover from bonking by stopping your exercise, eating quickly digestible carbohydrates, and waiting about 20–30 minutes for your blood sugar to return to normal.

There are no "good" or "bad" carbs. They are simply fuel for your body. Some carbohydrates, such as fruits and whole grains, contain vitamins, minerals, and fiber, which make them a good choice for overall health. Others, such as fruit juice and gummy candy, do not have useful nutrients other than the carbohydrate itself—but they are very useful in certain situations such as fueling active exercise.

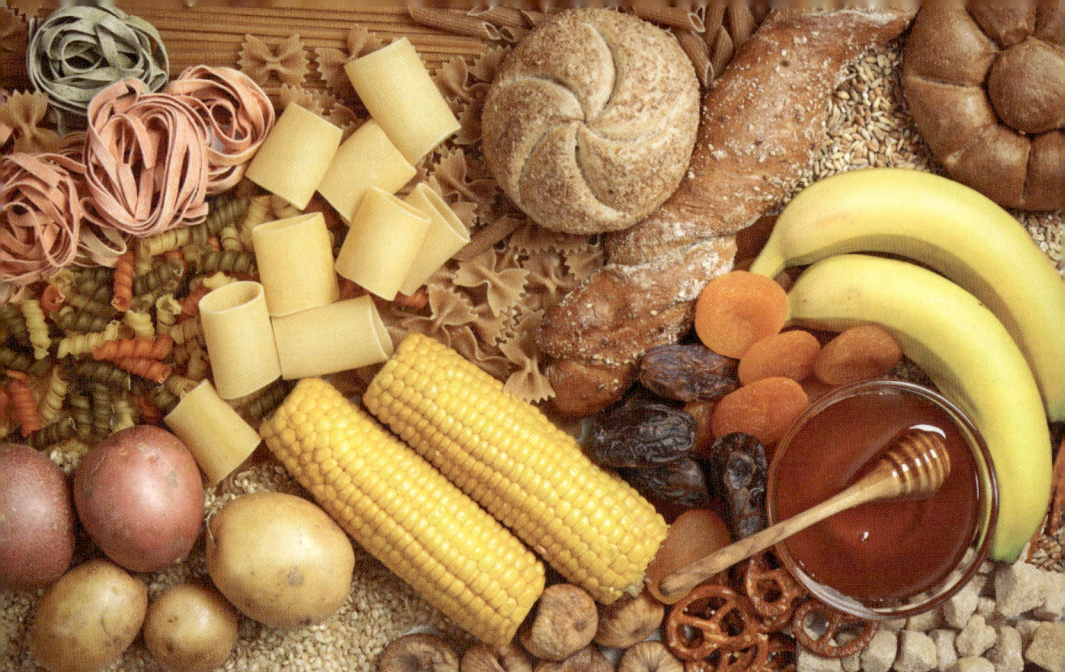

Eating regular meals helps regulate blood sugar. Eating before exercise if it's been more than 2 to 4 hours since your last meal can help you feel fueled and energized for the workout.

Food Sources of Carbohydrate
- Grains: rice, bread, pasta, oats, barley, cereal, etc.
- Fruit and fruit juice
- Starchy vegetables: potatoes, yams, sweet potatoes, squash, corn, peas
- Legumes and lentils: kidney beans, garbanzo beans, lima beans, etc.
- Sweets and desserts: candies, cookies, cake, soda (not diet)
- Milk and yogurt

Recommended Intake

Your carbohydrate needs may vary depending on your activity level. The baseline carbohydrate needs for normal healthy adults is around 3–5 grams per kilogram of body weight per day. If you are doing heavy training or have a long day of hiking, skiing, or climbing, you will need more carbohydrate, up to 7–12 grams per kilogram per day.

> **HOW TO CALCULATE YOUR WEIGHT IN KILOGRAMS**
>
> Take your weight in pounds and divide by 2.2.
>
> For example, a person weighing 170 pounds weighs 77.3 kg.
>
> 170 ÷ 2.2 = 77.3

8 NUTRITION FOR OUTDOOR RECREATION

PROTEIN

Role in the body: Protein plays several different roles in the body. It's an incredibly important nutrient for overall health and sports performance. It's involved with muscle growth and repair, bone health, immune function, tendon and ligament health, skin, and all organs.

Protein is made up of amino acids, which are like building blocks for protein. Some amino acids are not essential, meaning your body can manufacture them on its own. Some are essential, which means you need to get them in your diet in order for your body to operate at optimal health. Protein provides 4 calories per gram.

Eating a wide variety of foods usually supplies enough overall protein and amino acids. Those at risk for not getting enough protein are vegans, vegetarians, and people who are dieting or restricting their food intake.

Protein also helps people feel full and satisfied after a meal. Adequate protein is needed to help preserve lean muscle mass and rebuild and repair muscle tissue.

It is a crucial nutrient for athletes. Whether you are a climber, skier, hiker, alpinist, runner, or anything else, your body needs enough protein to perform optimally.

Food Sources of Protein
- Meat, fish, poultry
- Eggs
- Dairy products (milk, yogurt, cheese)
- Legumes (beans and lentils)
- Nuts and seeds
- Whole grains
- Soy products (tofu, tempeh, edamame)

In general, proteins from animal sources, such as eggs, meat, fish, poultry, and dairy products are better absorbed and used in your body than protein from plant sources (like tofu, beans, lentils, and nuts).

Protein from whole food sources offers a variety of nutrients. This is usually better than using a supplement such as a protein powder, although in some cases protein powders can be useful. See Chapter 4 for more information about supplements.

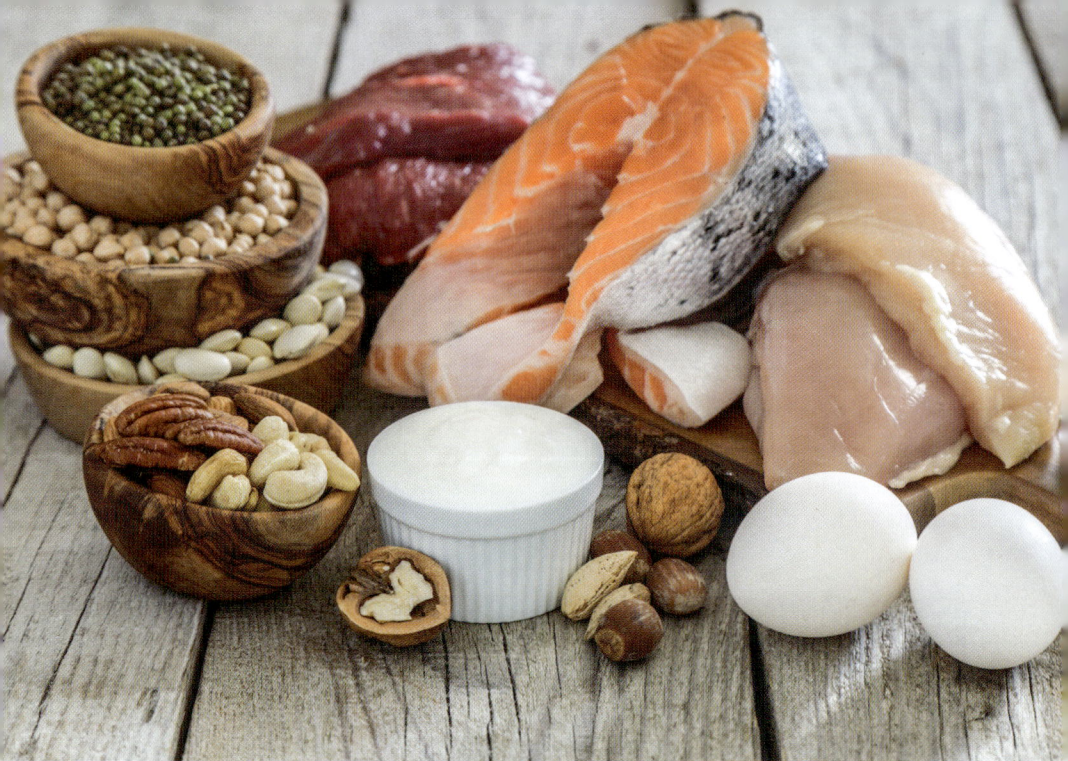

Recommended Intake

The amount of protein you may need varies widely based on your individual health history and your current exercise program. The minimum recommendation in the United States is 0.8 gram per kilogram per day.

Athletes will need much more to function optimally. Strength athletes and those undergoing a very intense training program may need 1.6–2.2 grams per kilogram per day, while an endurance athlete with a moderate training program may need around 1.2–1.6 grams per kilogram per day. If you are recovering from surgery or injury, you may also have increased protein needs, from about 1.3–2.0 grams per kilogram per day.

Find a qualified dietitian to help you determine your own calorie, protein, and carbohydrate needs for your particular situation.

FAT

Role in the body: Fat sometimes has a bad reputation, but fat is essential for life. Your body needs fat to absorb fat-soluble vitamins (vitamins A, D, E, and K). Fat makes up almost all cell membranes in the body. It also provides energy and essential fatty acids your body cannot do without. Fat provides 9 calories per gram.

Two main types of fats are saturated and unsaturated. In general, it's best to get most of your fat as unsaturated, as this is better for overall health and risk for heart disease. Foods like olive oil, fish, nuts, seeds, and avocado provide healthful fats that are beneficial for your body.

Fat also plays a role in energy metabolism. This means that fat can be a fuel source for your exercise and training. Fat is used as a fuel source, along with carbohydrate, when the body is exercising at a moderate intensity, such as jogging, walking, hiking, or skiing—anything you can do for several minutes to hours.

Food Sources of Fat
- Nuts and seeds
- Avocados
- Fish, meat, and poultry
- Eggs
- Olives
- Coconut
- Oils
- Full-fat dairy products, such as butter, yogurt, milk, cheese, and ice cream
- Fried foods, such as french fries, donuts, or breaded fried meat and fish
- Baked goods made with fat, such as biscuits, cakes, and cookies

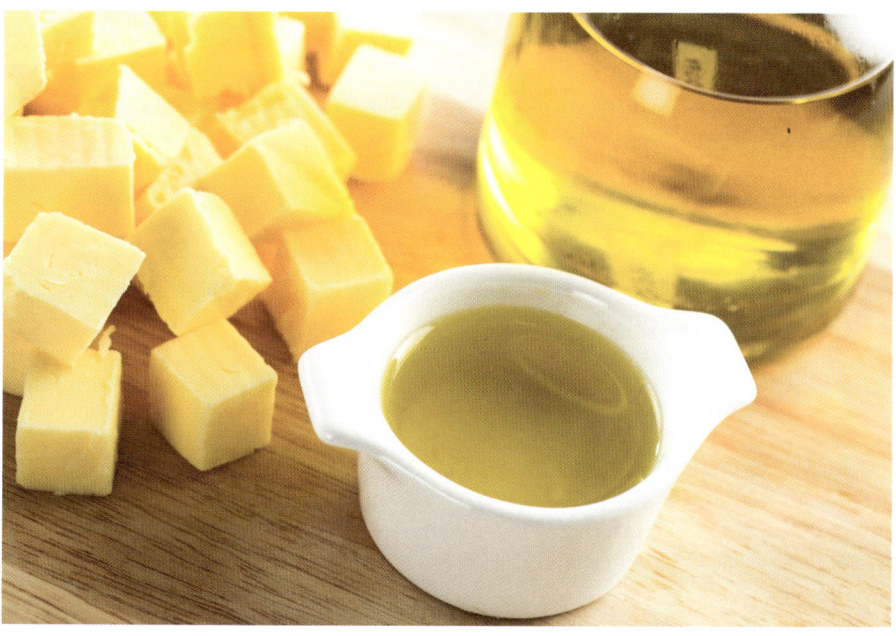

Recommended Intake

Most countries recommend limiting your intake to about 60–70 grams of fat per day, with 10 percent or less of total energy intake as saturated fat, and little to no trans fats.

ALCOHOL

Alcohol is technically a nutrient, as it provides energy at 7 calories per gram. However, it is not recommended to be a large part of your diet, as it is a toxin and can be very harmful to health.

Alcohol should be used only in moderation or not at all. Consult with your health care professional before using alcohol to ensure it will not interact with any medications or cause harm to your body.

While alcohol is not recommended, it is included here because many people drink it regularly. It's important to be aware of how it can affect your training. Alcohol can interfere with muscle rebuilding and repair after a training session, decrease concentration, interfere with quality sleep, dehydrate you, and decrease coordination. It can also add additional unwanted calories that your body may not need. Alcohol intake often thwarts your ability to eat a good meal if you are drinking instead of eating.

If you are a recreational athlete that wants to enjoy beer and pizza after a long hike, a couple of beers will likely be fine if you have no other health contraindications. Research around sports performance and alcohol suggest that a beer or two will not thwart training gains. However, binge drinking definitely can. If you are an elite or pro athlete, or have lofty training goals, consider omitting the alcohol because it won't do you any favors.

Also consider the safety aspects of alcohol. Refrain from drinking while doing your sport, so you can stay alert and aware in the backcountry, and follow proper safety protocol with a sharp mind (such as checking climbing knots). Save the alcohol for later.

Macronutrient	Calories per Gram	Main Food Sources	Function in Body	Intake Recommendations
Carbohydrate	4	Milk, yogurt, sweets/desserts, grains, fruits, starchy vegetables, legumes	Fuel most cells including brain and muscle; Regulate blood sugar	3–12 g/kg/day depending on activity level
Protein	4	Eggs, dairy, soy, meat, fish, whole grains	Repair and rebuild muscle tissue, organ tissue	1.2–2.0 g/kg/day depending on activity level and type
Fat	9	Meat, full-fat dairy, eggs, vegetable oil	Promote absorption of fat-soluble vitamins, cushion for organs, insulation for temperature regulation, hormone production	1 g/kg/day or no more than 20–30% of total calorie intake
Alcohol	7	Beer, wine, hard liquor, etc.	None; it is a toxin	None recommended

MICRONUTRIENTS

Micronutrients do not provide energy but play an important role in health and body functions. There are many micronutrients; only the main ones will be discussed here.

Guidelines from the National Institutes of Health (NIH) (United States) recommend intakes for most adults age 18 and older. You may need a different amount based on your health history. Always check with your doctor before taking any vitamin, mineral, or supplement.

Please note that the reference table below is based on NIH information, which only lists males and females. Since there is no data on nonbinary and trans persons, it is not listed. For a general recommendation, you may assume your needs may line up with your gender assigned at birth, but be sure to talk with your doctor about your specific needs.

1 / NUTRITION BASICS   13

Most people do not need multivitamins or single micronutrient supplements. If you can eat a wide variety of foods, you are likely able to get all you need from your diet. However, some situations may need extra supplementation, such as iron deficiency anemia or vitamin D deficiency.

If you suspect a nutrient deficiency, test—don't guess! Ask your doctor for a blood draw to check for specific deficiencies. It is not smart to take a supplement if you're not sure if you really need it, or what dose or form to take it. Nutrient toxicities can occur.

Some people who may need to supplement are vegans (with vitamin B12), those with a known nutrient deficiency, and those with gastrointestinal concerns.

Micronutrient	Function in the Body	Food Sources	Recommended Intake per Day
Iron	Carries oxygen to tissues, helps with metabolism and cell function	Meat, seafood, nuts, beans, dark leafy vegetables, fortified cereals and breads	Males 8 mg, Females 18 mg
Calcium	Bone health and strength, nerve conduction, enzyme and hormone function, muscle contraction	Dairy products, fish with edible bones (sardines), kale, broccoli, fortified soy and cereal products	1,000 mg, 1,200 mg for females age 51+
Zinc	Helps with numerous cell functions, immunity, growth in children	Fortified cereals, meat, poultry, beans, nuts, seafood, dairy products	Males 8 mg, Females 11 mg
Magnesium	Enzyme reactions, muscle contraction, blood pressure regulation, bone health	Meat, poultry, eggs, fruit, leafy green vegetables, fortified cereals	Males 420 mg, Females 320 mg
Potassium	Heartbeat, nerve conduction, blood pressure regulation	Meat, milk, fruits, vegetables, legumes, whole grains	4.7 g

Micronutrient	Function in the Body	Food Sources	Recommended Intake per Day
Vitamin A	Immunity, vision, eye health, skin health, bone growth	Liver, milk, eggs, leafy vegetables, carrots, sweet potatoes, broccoli, squash, cantaloupe	Males 900 mcg Retinal Activity Equivalents (RAE), Females 700 mcg RAE
Vitamin E	Antioxidant, immunity, cell function	Vegetable oils, nuts, spinach, broccoli, fortified foods (often used as a preservative)	15 mg
Vitamin D	Nerve function, muscle function, bone health, immunity	Fortified foods, fatty fish, egg yolks, mushrooms. Also synthesized in your skin when in the sun.	15 mcg
Vitamin K	Blood clotting, bone health	Green leafy vegetables, vegetable oil, meat, cheese, eggs, soybeans	Males 120 mcg, Females 90 mcg
Vitamin C	Antioxidant, iron absorption, immunity, skin health	Citrus fruits, bell peppers, kiwi, broccoli, berries, potatoes, tomatoes, cantaloupe	Males 90 mg, Females 75 mg
Vitamin B6	Enzyme reactions, metabolism, immunity, fetal brain development	Poultry, fish, potatoes, fruit, legumes, soy products, bananas, watermelon	1.3 mg
Vitamin B12	Nerve and cell function, DNA production	Liver, clams, fish, meat, poultry, nutritional yeast, fortified cereal	2.4 mcg

(*continued*)

Micronutrient	Function in the Body	Food Sources	Recommended Intake per Day
Riboflavin	Cell function, energy metabolism	Eggs, meat, milk, asparagus, broccoli, spinach, fortified cereal	Males 1.3 mg, Females 1.1 mg
Thiamine	Energy metabolism, nerve function	Meat, fish, pork, whole grains, fortified cereal	Males 1.2 mg, Females 1.1 mg
Niacin	Energy metabolism, cell function	Meat, fish, poultry, nuts, legumes, whole grains, fortified cereal	Males 16 mg Niacin Equivalents (NE), Females 14 mg NE
Biotin	Energy metabolism, skin/hair/nail health	Meat, fish, eggs, nuts and seeds, sweet potatoes, spinach, broccoli	30 mcg
Folate	Cell metabolism, DNA production	Liver, fortified cereal, leafy green vegetables, fruit, nuts, legumes, peas	400 mcg

FLUIDS

Fluids are very important for outdoor recreation. Improper hydration can lead to medical emergencies and even death.

Fluids are key to proper body functions. Fluids help regulate temperature, lubricate joints, carry oxygen and nutrients to the cells, and excrete toxins via urine, sweat, and stool.

Here's the good news: Any fluid except alcohol can "count" toward your hydration needs. Yup, even coffee! Many fruits and vegetables have a high water content as well. Oranges, apples, watermelon, cucumber, and more can help contribute toward total body hydration.

What causes water loss in the first place? The body is naturally always trying to achieve a homeostatic state. This means it is trying to optimize fluid balance, as well as eliminate waste products and maintain blood electrolyte levels. We drink in response to thirst, the body uses the fluid and excretes what it doesn't need, and the cycle begins again.

Fluid loss can be increased for many reasons:

- Diarrhea/vomiting
- Excess sweating
- High altitude (increased loss in respiration as well as increased diuresis)
- Flying on a plane (the cabin is dry and respiration losses increase)
- Heat/humidity
- Some medications

DEHYDRATION

Dehydration is something you don't want to mess with, especially in the backcountry. Most sports nutrition literature lists clinical dehydration as losing more than 2 percent of your body weight within a short time.

Here are some signs and symptoms of dehydration:

- Dark, smelly, or concentrated urine
- Decreased performance
- Increased rate of perceived exertion
- Dizziness
- Thirst
- Lightheadedness
- Rapid heartbeat
- Lethargy or sleepiness
- Nausea and/or vomiting

Read that list again. Imagine you are far from any cell signal, and you are in the middle of your favorite outdoor activity. Let's say it's rock climbing. Now imagine trying to climb when you feel dizzy, lightheaded, lethargic, and nauseated. Could you do a proper safety check while tying your knots? Would you have the strength to climb upwards? Could you manage an emergency situation, like an unexpected rock fall? Probably not very well.

Hydration is crucial. Look for urine that is light yellow (like straw or lemonade color). If it is dark like tea or cola, you are dehydrated. Seek medical attention immediately.

OVERHYDRATION

Believe it or not, you can become overly hydrated. People may drink too much if they are worried about hydration, they are going very slowly for long distances (because there is more opportunity to drink and less chance of losing it in sweat at a lower-intensity pace), or they have a medical condition that causes them to retain water (such as a kidney or heart condition).

Overhydration can also be called hyponatremia, which means a dilution of blood sodium. This can occur if you drink too much fluid. A secondary driver may be inadequate sodium (a key electrolyte) intake in your fluids or food.

Some signs and symptoms of overhydration include:

- Headache
- Dizziness
- Confusion
- Nausea and/or vomiting
- Lethargy
- Muscle weakness, spasms, or cramps

Since some of these symptoms also match up with dehydration, you can troubleshoot which is the cause of your symptoms by considering them in the context of your day. If you were drinking a lot of water on a very hot day and started feeling these symptoms, you may need to add some sodium or electrolytes (sodium is the primary electrolyte lost in sweat). If you feel these symptoms but have not drunk much, or it is coupled with low urine output and dark, concentrated urine, you know you are dehydrated.

A general rule of thumb for most workout scenarios is to drink 8–16 ounces every 60 minutes. You can use this as a starting point for adequate hydration, but then dial in more specifically for your individual situation.

CALCULATING SWEAT RATE

Here's how to find out your individual sweat rate. People have different sweat rates, so a one-size-fits-all approach to hydration isn't effective, and thirst isn't always a reliable indicator of fluid needs.

SWEAT RATE CHEAT SHEET

1. Empty your bladder.
2. Weigh yourself with as little clothing as possible before your workout. My weight is _____ pounds.
3. Do your normal workout. Do not eat or urinate. Drink as usual. Work out for 1 hour.
4. Keep track of how much you drank during your workout. I drank _____ ounces during my workout.
5. Towel off any sweat. Weigh yourself in as little clothing as possible after your workout. I weigh _____ pounds after my workout.
6. Pre-workout weight _____ – post-workout weight _____ = _____ pounds. _____ pounds × 16 = _____ oz.
7. _____ ounces consumed during my workout + _____ = _____ my sweat rate in ounces per hour.
8. Repeat this at least 2 more times under similar circumstances (temperature, altitude, humidity) to find your average sweat rate. When you work out, drink _____ oz per hour.

1. Weigh yourself nude before a workout.
2. Work out for about 60 minutes (don't pee!).
3. Keep track of how much you drink during the workout.
4. Weigh yourself after the workout (nude again).
5. Calculate how many pounds you lost: For every pound of weight you lost, you need to drink 16–24 ounces of fluid. If you drank fluid during the workout, add that to your total weight lost (more than a 2 percent body weight loss is considered clinical dehydration).

For example, if you lost 2 pounds but also drank 16 ounces (1 pound), you know the scale would have shown that you lost 3 pounds (not 2) if you had not drunk anything. This means you lose 3 pounds of fluids in a 60-minute workout. The next time you work out, you know you can drink about 48 ounces (3 pounds × 16 ounces per pound) to minimize fluid loss.

A question you may have while reading this is: Do I need to *exactly* replace my fluid losses? That sounds like a lot to drink in 1 hour!

> There is a really cool online calculator at sweatratecalculator.com. It can only calculate for running and cycling, but it does take into account variables such as your body weight, outside temperature, humidity, wind speed, and more. It is a good resource if you want to get an estimated sweat rate.

The answer is no, you don't. You want to drink enough to avoid dehydration, or greater than 2 percent body weight lost over the course of the workout.

For a short session, say, 1 hour of surfing, you don't need to overthink your hydration strategy. Just start your session well hydrated and drink afterward.

For longer excursions, like a multi-day backpacking trip, it becomes more important to closely replace fluid losses day over day to maintain adequate hydration and stay safe.

Remember that sweat rate can change based on circumstances, such as temperature, altitude, and humidity. Just measuring your sweat rate one time will not give you an accurate picture across all scenarios, but it can help you get a snapshot of what is going on. An estimated sweat rate is better than not knowing how much your body sweat losses are.

ELECTROLYTES/SPORTS DRINKS

Sports drinks sometimes get a bad rap. Due to their sugar and salt content, some people feel they should steer clear. However, added sugar and salt are exactly the point! There's a large body of evidence that shows simple sugars (those lovely carbohydrates) help with sports performance, as carbs are a main energy source for working muscles. Salt in the form of sodium chloride is the main electrolyte lost in sweat. Using a sports drink is a smart way to deliver fluid, electrolytes, and fuel to the body all in one product.

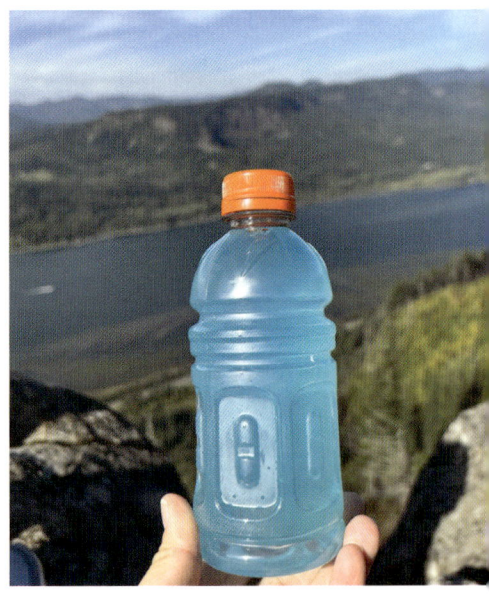

NUTRITION FOR OUTDOOR RECREATION

Some situations where you may need a sports drink:

- You want to rely on it for some calories/fuel.
- You need electrolytes.
- You like the taste and it helps you keep hydrated.
- You drink it after a long, hard workout to rehydrate.

Some situations where you might need to avoid using a sports drink:

- It is too heavy or cumbersome to carry a packaged drink or sports drink powder.
- You get diarrhea or gastrointestinal upset when using a sports drink.
- You are not exercising for very long (less than 90 minutes) and are going into the workout well hydrated and fueled.

Ingredients in Sports Drinks	Examples	Purpose	Notes
Electrolytes	Sodium, potassium, magnesium	Fluid balance; prevention of dehydration and hyponatremia	Sodium is the main ingredient lost in sweat. The other electrolytes are less important. People lose between ~200 and 1,500 mg of sodium per hour.
Carbohydrates	Glucose, fructose, maltodextrin	Easily digestible fuel for the working muscles during long or intense workouts	Aim for minimum of 30 g of carbs per hour (from food, fluids, or both).
Vitamins	B vitamins, vitamin C	Some vitamins are involved in energy metabolism.	In a sports drink they are just a marketing gimmick.
Extras	Amino acids, taurine, caffeine, B vitamins	Caffeine can improve performance, time to fatigue, and cognition. See Chapter 4 for more on supplements.	With the exception of caffeine, most ingredients are a marketing gimmick to make the drink seem more effective.

WAYS TO CARRY FLUIDS

You may have your own system for fluid intake. If so, that's great! If not, here are some ideas. These have different applications depending on which adventure you are doing.

- Camelbak or other bladder/hose system integrated into your backpack
- Running vests with built-in pockets for water bottles
- Handheld water bottle with sleeve to hook over hand while running or hiking
- Nalgene, Hydroflask, Stanley, Yeti, etc. water bottles
- Collapsible plastic or silicone bladders or "bottles"
- Water filter/purifier or LifeStraw for outdoor activities of long duration near a natural water source

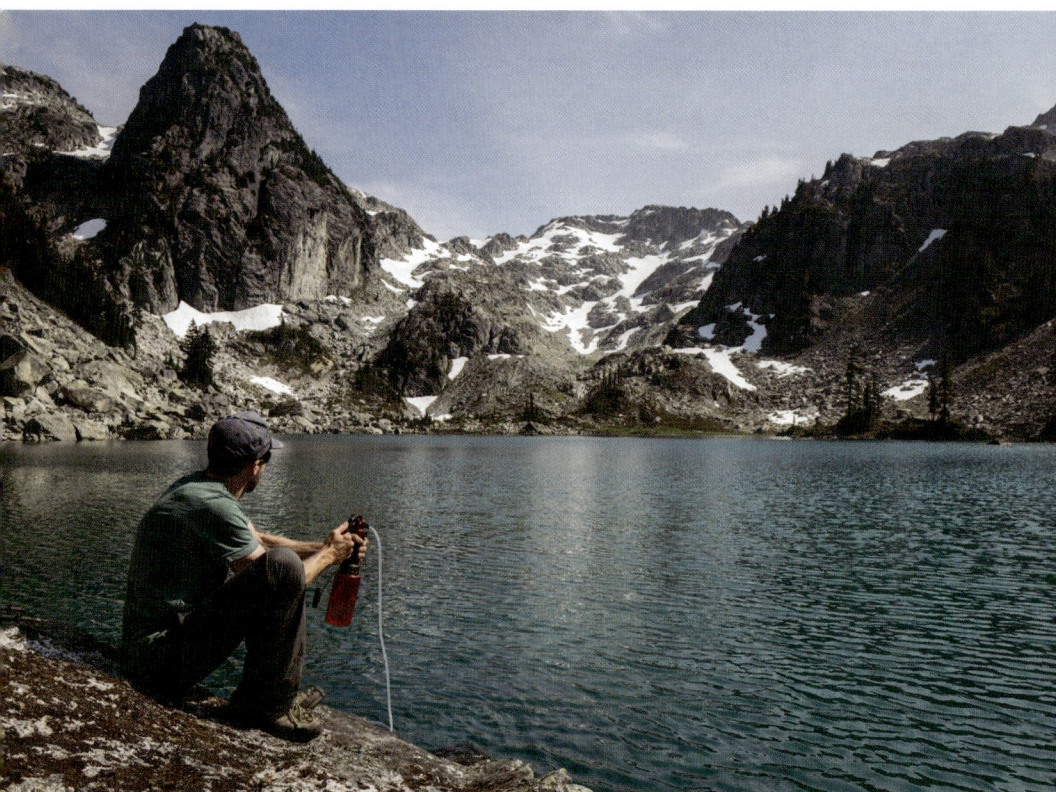

THE WRAP-UP
Worthy nutrition goals include:

- Eat enough to support basic body processes.
- Eat enough to support training and movement (before, during, and after activity).
- Eat a healthful diet made of mostly whole grains, fruits/vegetables, nuts/seeds, dairy products, and lean protein.
- Refuel and rehydrate after workouts to promote recovery.
- Maintain a good relationship with food, body, and sport.

These goals can be supported by eating enough calories and macronutrients in your overall diet. Eating a variety of foods including fruits, vegetables, nuts/seeds, whole grains, lean protein, and healthful fats can support an overall outdoor athlete's health. Understanding your specific fueling and hydration needs will help you feel fueled and energized for whatever activity you are doing.

REFERENCES

Burke, L. M., and V. Deakin. *Clinical Sports Nutrition*, 5th Ed. McGraw-Hill Education, 2015.

Burke, L. M., J. A. Hawley, S. H. Wong, and A. E. Jeukendrup. "Carbohydrates for Training and Competition." *Journal of Sports Sciences* 29, suppl. 1 (2011), S17–S27.

Cotter, J. D., S. N. Thornton, J. K. W. Lee, and P. B. Laursen. "Are We Being Drowned in Hydration Advice? Thirsty for More?" *Extreme Physiology & Medicine* 3, no. 18 (2014).

Gorissen, S. H., and O. C. Witard. "Characterising the Muscle Anabolic Potential of Dairy, Meat and Plant-Based Protein Sources in Older Adults." *Conference on "Nutrition and Exercise for Health and Performance" Symposium 2: Maintenance of Muscle Mass for Healthy Ageing*, 2017.

Hawley, J. A. "Fat Adaptation Science: Low-Carbohydrate, High-Fat Diets to Alter Fuel Utilization and Promote Training Adaptation." *Nestle Nutrition Institute Workshop* 69 (2011), 59–77.

Maughan, R. J. *The Biochemical Basis of Sports Performance*. Oxford, UK: Oxford University Press, 2010.

National Institutes of Health, Offices of Dietary Supplements, Vitamin and Mineral Supplement Fact Sheets, 2023.

Phillips, S. M. "Dietary Protein Requirements and Adaptive Advantages in Athletes." *British Journal of Nutrition* 108 (2012), S158–S167.

"Position of the Academy of Nutrition and Dietetics, Dietitians of Canada, and the American College of Sports Medicine: Nutrition and Athletic Performance." *Journal of the Academy of Nutrition and Dietetics* 116 (2016), 501–28.

Schoenfeld, B. J., and A. A. Aragon. "How Much Protein Can the Body Use in a Single Meal for Muscle-Building? Implications for Daily Protein Distribution." *Journal of the International Society of Sports Nutrition* 15, no. 10 (2018).

Trexler, E. T., A. E. Smith-Ryan, and L. E. Norton. "Metabolic Adaptation to Weight Loss: Implications for the Athlete." *Journal of the International Society of Sports Nutrition* 11, no. 1 (February 27, 2014), 7. doi: 10.1186/1550-2783-11-7. PMID: 24571926; PMCID: PMC3943438.

2
MEAL PLANNING, NUTRIENT TIMING, AND NUTRITION PERIODIZATION

John is a busy guy. He wakes up early to exercise, then showers quickly and goes to work. He usually has a cup of coffee in the morning, and a salad for lunch. By dinnertime, he is ravenous. He is concerned about his nightly snacks, where he eats ice cream, chips, candy, popcorn, and anything else in the house. He feels he may have a bingeing problem. What he really has is a meal timing problem!

His body is not getting enough food or nutrients throughout the day, so it's asking for a lot at night. What feels like uncontrollable cravings is actually a biological response to food deprivation. Once John can eat a full breakfast, lunch, and dinner, his large cravings disappear.

This is one example of how meal planning and nutrient timing can help support someone's overall health and performance.

Now that you have some nutrition basics laying your foundation of knowledge, let's talk about nutrient timing. In this chapter, we will cover:

- The plate method for easy/moderate/hard days
- How to calculate your own nutrient needs
- Nutrient timing for pre-, during, and post-workout
- Periodization for day to day, training blocks, and overall year

Remember the key points from Chapter 1. This chapter is designed to help you meet these goals:

- Eat enough to support basic body processes.
- Eat enough to support training and movement (before, during, and after activity).
- Eat a healthful diet made of mostly whole grains, fruits/vegetables, nuts/seeds, dairy products, and lean protein.
- Refuel and rehydrate after workouts to promote recovery.
- Maintain a good relationship with food, body, and sport.

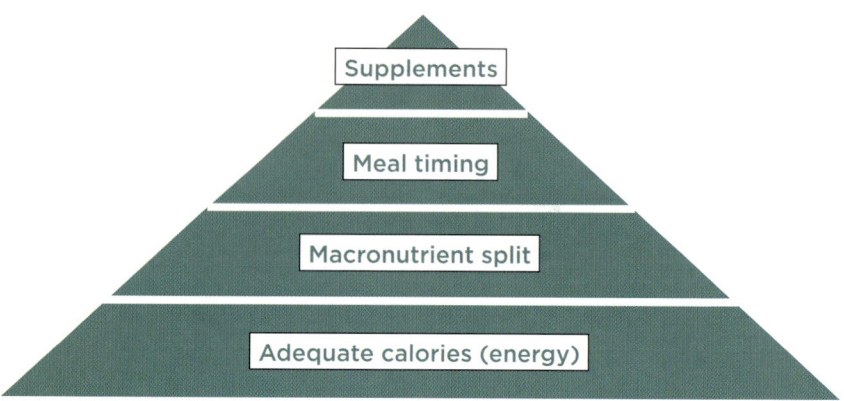

When thinking about sports performance, there is a hierarchy of nutrition principles. This chapter will talk about the bottom three concepts. For more on supplements, see Chapter 4.

THE PLATE METHOD

Before we get into the details of how to estimate your energy and macronutrient needs, let's first learn the plate method. This is my favorite method of understanding how to eat, because it is so simple to implement. You just imagine a dinner plate, and divide your food groups like a pie chart as seen on the next page.

This method ensures you get the approximate macro split and calorie level appropriate for your training load that day without having to weigh or measure food, or count calories and macros.

Extras like condiments and drinks can be added according to your own taste preferences. Fat is not listed as part of the pie chart, because it is usually inherent in foods and doesn't have to be added. For example, if your protein item on your plate is beef, there is going to be some fat in that beef. Similarly, if your carbohydrate item is pasta, you may put some pesto on it, which has fat in it. Many people sauté vegetables in oil, or put dressing on a salad, so they get their fat intake without having to think about adding it.

LIGHT TRAINING DAY

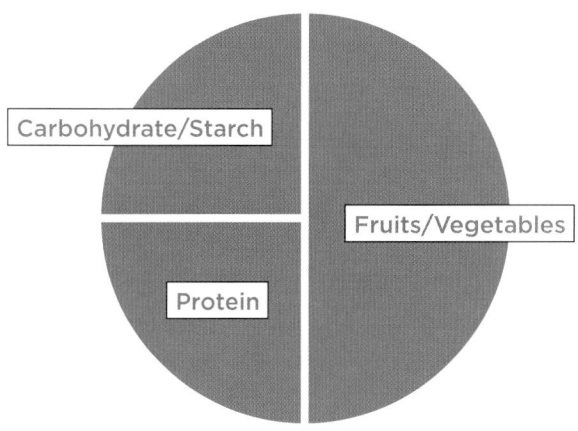

MODERATE TRAINING DAY

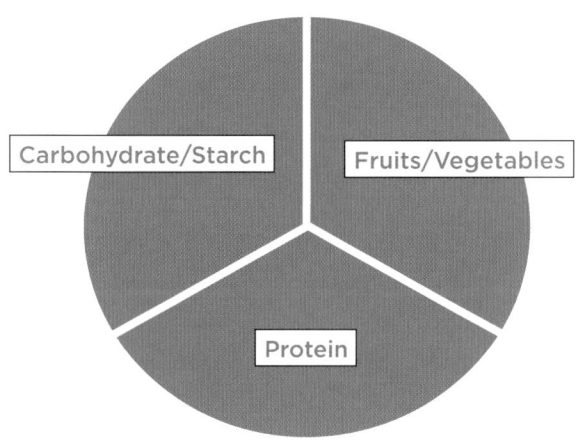

HEAVY TRAINING DAY

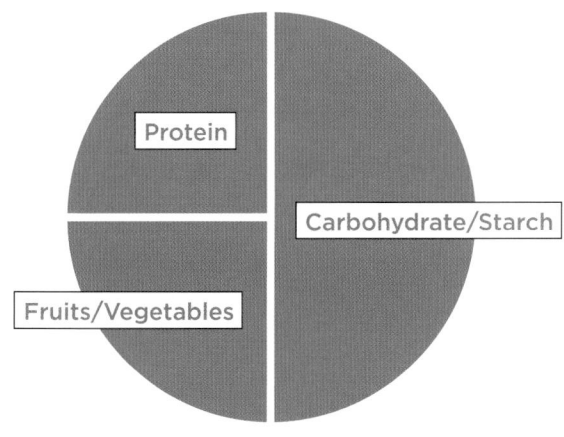

HOW TO CALCULATE YOUR OWN NUTRIENT NEEDS

If you don't want to use the plate method and want something a bit more specific, you can use a variety of options to calculate energy needs.

First, it is important to get enough overall calories (energy). This is the basis of your diet—the bottom of the pyramid. Eating enough can help support not only the basic body processes, such as digestion, heart rate, and respiration—but also supports the training and adventuring as well as recovery. For more on this, see Chapter 6 where we talk about relative energy deficiency in sport.

HOW TO CALCULATE ENERGY NEEDS

The Energy Availability Method

The general recommendation is to eat 30–45 calories per kilogram of fat-free mass per day. (Note: 30 kcal/kg/day is on the low end and 45 kcal/kg/day is for optimal energy availability.) For this calculation, you need to know your body composition.

Let's say you weigh 170 pounds and have 20 percent body fat.

1. Convert pounds to kilograms (kg) by dividing by 2.2; 170 ÷ 2.2 = 77.2 kg.
2. Find your fat-free mass; 20 percent × 77.2 kg (or 0.20 × 77.2) = 15.4 kg of fat. 77.2 total body weight minus 15.4 kg of fat = 61.8 kg fat-free mass.
3. 61.8 kg fat-free mass × 30 to 45 calories/kg = *1,854–2,781 calories* needed daily to have adequate energy availability (you may need more calories than this, depending on your activity level).

The Predictive Equation Methods

There are several equations available to calculate estimated energy needs. All have their pros and cons, and all have a margin of error. It is easy to find online calculators for these equations.

Some common ones are:

- Mifflin-St. Jeor equation
    Females: (10*weight [kg]) + (6.25*height [cm]) – (5*age [years]) – 161
    Males: (10*weight [kg]) + (6.25*height [cm]) – (5*age [years]) + 5

- Schofield equation
    Females: 13.623W + 2.83H + 98.2
    Males 15.057W − 0.1H + 705.8

- Harris Benedict equation
    Females: (9.5634 × weight in kg) + (1.8496 × height in cm) − (4.6756 × age in years) + 655.0955
    Males: (13.7516 × weight in kg) + (.0033 × height in cm) − (6.755 × age in years) + 66.473

These equations give you a baseline—the minimum amount of energy your body needs to maintain body processes. From there, you need to multiply by an activity factor to determine your overall calorie needs. Activity factors vary slightly, but usually fall within the following ranges:

Sedentary	1.2–1.3
Lightly active	1.375–1.45
Moderately active	1.55–1.65
Active	1.725–1.85
Very active	1.9–2.2

You use these activity factors by determining your basic energy needs through one of the above equations, then multiply by the activity factor. For example, if you plug in your data into the Mifflin-St. Jeor equation and discover that your needs are 1,500 calories per day, you then multiply 1,500 by 1.55 if you are a "moderately active" person: 1,500 × 1.55 = 2,325 calories needed daily.

The METS Method

METS stands for metabolic equivalents. One MET is the amount of energy your body uses in 1 minute while resting (measured in calories). Light activities are less than 3 METS (like easy walking). Moderate activities are 3–6 METS, such as brisk walking or moderate exercise. Intense activities are over 6 METS, like walking uphill while carrying a loaded backpack, or cross-country skiing.

You can use METS to estimate how many calories you burn during an exercise. This would not help you determine your overall daily calorie needs, but can help you understand the energy cost of a particular exercise so you can fuel appropriately. Here is the equation:

$$\text{Exercise calories} = (\text{MET level of activity} \times 3.5 \times \text{weight (kg)} \times \text{minutes of activity}) / 200$$

Here is an example of a cross-country skier (9.0 METS) who weighs 70 kilograms and skis for 3 hours.

$$(9.0 \text{ METS} \times 3.5 \times 70\text{kg} \times 180 \text{ minutes}) / 200 = 1{,}985$$
calories used while cross-country skiing (wow!)

But you may have another question . . . Can I just rely on what my Garmin/Apple Watch/smart device tells me?

Kind of, but not really.

These devices can get you in the ballpark, but they are notorious for being inaccurate as far as measuring calories burned. Some can be off by up to 40 percent! That is a big deal when you are trying to understand your own energy needs. Similarly, if you are tracking food intake on an app, these also

CALORIE TRACKING

Calorie tracking can be useful for some, and disordered for others.

How can you know if you should track calories?

Helpful Tracking	Disordered Tracking
Feels empowering	Feels tedious or obsessive
Gives useful information to meet goals	You feel guilt or shame if you go over your calorie goals
Flexibility in diet and exercise is preserved	You feel anxious if you do not track one day
You are willing to not track for a day or two	Tracking disrupts hunger or fullness cues
You are ok with eating out or special food occasions such as birthdays	You skip holidays or birthday celebrations because you can't track accurately
You can honor hunger/fullness cues	

have a margin of error. These tools can be useful but be sure to take the numbers with a grain of salt.

MACRONUTRIENTS (CARBOHYDRATES, PROTEIN, AND FAT)

The next most important consideration is how your macronutrients are distributed from meal to meal and day to day. This is sometimes called your macronutrient (or "macro") split. The plate method mentioned above can help guide your macronutrient split. Or you could calculate your particular needs. For this information, keep reading!

Carbohydrates

Carbohydrate needs vary based on the type, duration, and intensity of the activity. Since carbohydrate is your muscle and brain's preferred energy source, it is essential to get enough both overall to support day-to-day recovery, and within the exercise itself.

Carbohydrates are a key macronutrient involved with your outdoor sports performance. Whether you are skiing, hiking, climbing, biking, or anything else—carbohydrates are crucial to help you feel and perform your best. They can also help with low blood sugar and bonking. I am continually amazed by my clients who, when they learn to understand how much carbohydrate they need, can feel so much better! They can feel more energized, have better focus, and experience increased motivation.

For easy to moderate days, like a 60-minute jog or gym session, you only need about 3–5 grams per kilogram of carbohydrate. For more intense days, such as backpacking with elevation gain and carrying a pack, you will need closer to 10–12 grams per kilogram of carbohydrate for those days.

CARB NEEDS FOR TRAINING

Daily Training

Light Activity	Moderate Activity	High Activity	Very High Activity
3-5 g/kg/day	5-7 g/kg/day	6-10 g/kg/day	8-12 g/kg/day

During Exercise

0-60 Minutes	60-120 Minutes	Over 2 Hours
None needed	30 g/hour	60-90 g/hour

CARBOHYDRATE ABSORPTION

If you've ever chugged a concentrated sports drink and then experienced bloating, sloshy stomach, cramping, or diarrhea, you know what it feels like to overload your gut. Your small intestine can only absorb so much carbohydrate at one time. Think of the hollow part of your small intestine like a river, and the intestinal wall is the banks of the river. There are little ferry boats that can take the carbohydrate molecule, like glucose or fructose, from the river to the banks to move it into your bloodstream. But there are only so many ferries! And some ferries only fit glucose molecules, and some only fit fructose molecules. If there are too many carbohydrate molecules, it just creates a traffic jam and gastrointestinal distress. This is why training your gut, practicing your fueling, and using multiple forms of carbohydrate can help alleviate any stomach issues and help you feel well fueled.

Here is a list of simple carbs you can use while exercising:

Exercise Fueling Guide

1 oz. pretzels: 23 g carbs
1 banana: 27 g
1 white mini-bagel: 23 g
8 oz sports drink: 14 g
1 orange: 11 g
1 fruit leather: 11 g
1 apple: 25 g
1 applesauce pouch: 15 g
1 oz animal crackers: 21 g
½ c blueberries: 21 g
1 graham cracker sheet: 11 g
½ c dried apricots: 40 g
1 c grapes: 16 g
15 crackers: 10 g
1 box raisins: 34 g
1 c chocolate milk: 26 g

1 c Chex: 26 B
1 c Rice Krispies: 21 g
1 c corn flakes: 24 g
6 sports chews: 24 g
2 rice cakes: 14 g
1 pouch fruit snacks: 21 g
1 packet honey: 12 g
1 sports gel: 22 g
2 dates: 36 g
1 baked potato: 37 g
19 Swedish fish: 35 g
1 white roll: 16 g
1 Pop Tart: 36 g
½ c white rice ball: 22 g
1 Rice Krispie treat: 17 g
Jam sandwich on white bread: 50 g

A basic rule of thumb is to eat at least 30 grams of carbohydrate per hour of exercise. You may need more than this. If your workout is intense, at high altitude, or a very long duration, you may need more like 60–90 grams per hour. For example, a moderate day hike may need 30–60 grams per hour, but an off-road 100-mile mountain biking race may need 60–90 grams per hour.

Some athletes have been successful eating up to 100–120 grams per hour of carbohydrate. The longer the duration and the more intense the exercise, the more carbohydrate demands increase. Multi-stage cycling tour riders, ultra-runners, and the like can train their guts to tolerate this level of carbohydrate, and they often find success with faster times and less fatigue.

Pro tips to make your carb intake a success:

- Avoid foods high in fat, fiber, or protein during active intense exercise. Aim for less than 9 grams of fat, 4 grams of fiber, and 4 grams of protein in your food item.
- Aim for simple carbohydrate foods. These are easy on the stomach and digested quickly to fuel the muscles fast.
- If you need 60–100+ grams per hour, use mixed fuel sources. For example, don't use just gels with one carbohydrate source. Use a gel with multiple sources, or multiple foods. This is because the body can only absorb up to about 60 grams of glucose per hour. If you use only glucose, the transporters in the intestine that help absorb the glucose will be overwhelmed, resulting in cramping, diarrhea, or bloating. But using different fuels like fructose allows multiple transporters to function at the same time, thereby being able to deliver a high amount of carbohydrate without overwhelming your gut. Note: Many sports products are designed to have the optimal ratio of glucose to fructose.

Protein

The Recommended Daily Allowance for protein in the United States is 0.8 gram per kilogram per day (g/kg/day).

This is enough to survive, not enough to optimize sports performance and recovery. An outdoor athlete needs much more.

In general, about 1.2–2.0 grams/kilogram/day is needed for outdoor athletes. The lower end of the range is recommended for general light-to-moderate activity level. The higher end is for a fat loss phase, power endurance phase, or strength-training phase.

Protein is best utilized in the body by spreading out an even intake of protein throughout the day. Aim for 20–40 grams of protein at each meal, with 3–4 meals per day and 1–3 snacks depending on your own energy needs and hunger levels.

To give you an idea of what to eat, the following foods contain about 20 grams of protein:

- 4 oz chicken breast
- 3 large eggs
- 1 cup cottage cheese
- 1 cup tofu
- 3 oz steak
- 10 oz cooked kidney beans

Fat

Unfortunately, there is not a lot of research on fat needs for athletes. We don't have any fancy equations to estimate your fat needs. The general recommendation at this time is to aim for at least 1 gram/kilogram/day. Usually, athletes get enough fat in their diet without having to think about it or track it. Since fat is common in many foods and cooking preparation methods (such as using olive oil to sauté vegetables), it isn't a macronutrient that needs a lot of attention.

Some people try to limit their fat when they are in a fat loss phase and aiming for a calorie deficit. This is because fat is the most "expensive" macronutrient at 9 calories per gram (as compared to 4 calories per gram for carbohydrate and protein). This strategy works for some. For others, it feels restrictive and unsatisfying. You can experiment with fat intake and find what works for you. Just be sure to get enough. A very lowfat diet (less than 10 percent of overall calories) can lead to negative health outcomes.

* * *

If you have any special dietary needs related to a medical condition, such as diabetes or high cholesterol, check with your doctor and dietitian for more specific guidance.

EASY MEAL IDEAS

First, have some ingredients on hand that could be easily gathered to make a meal.

- Pre-washed salad greens
- Chicken: pre-cooked bites, rotisserie, grilled breast, canned, etc.
- Canned or pouch tuna or salmon
- Frozen veggies and fruit
- Easy veggies: baby carrots, grape tomatoes, olives, baby bell peppers
- Tofu cubes
- Canned beans: black, chickpea, etc.
- Pre-seasoned pouches of lentils (I like the Tasty Bites brand)
- Boiled eggs
- Rice or quinoa
- Nuts
- Cheese
- Russet potatoes (bake a batch of 5–7 at once)
- Steel cut oats

Next, make your meal!

These ingredients are designed to be gathered quickly for a nourishing meal that doesn't take too much cooking or prep.

Add side dishes like fruit, a smoothie, a roll, or anything else to round out your meal. Here are some meals you can make with your ingredients:

Copycat Chick-Fil-A salad: Greens + tomato + carrots + chicken nuggets + boiled egg

Southwest grain bowl: Quinoa + frozen corn + black beans + rotisserie chicken shreds + salsa

Lentil bowl: Rice + lentils with a side salad

Charcuterie: Fresh veggies (olives + carrots + grape tomatoes) + cheese cubes + crackers + nuts + boiled egg + deli meat

Tuna or tofu salad: Tuna or tofu on a bed of greens + chopped peppers

Loaded baked potato: Potato + lentils + cheese with a side salad

Savory oats: Oatmeal + nuts + egg

Sweet oats: Oatmeal + frozen berries + nuts

These are just some ideas. Add your own, or use this list to go grocery shopping and have these ingredients on hand. Then you'll have quick meals all week long!

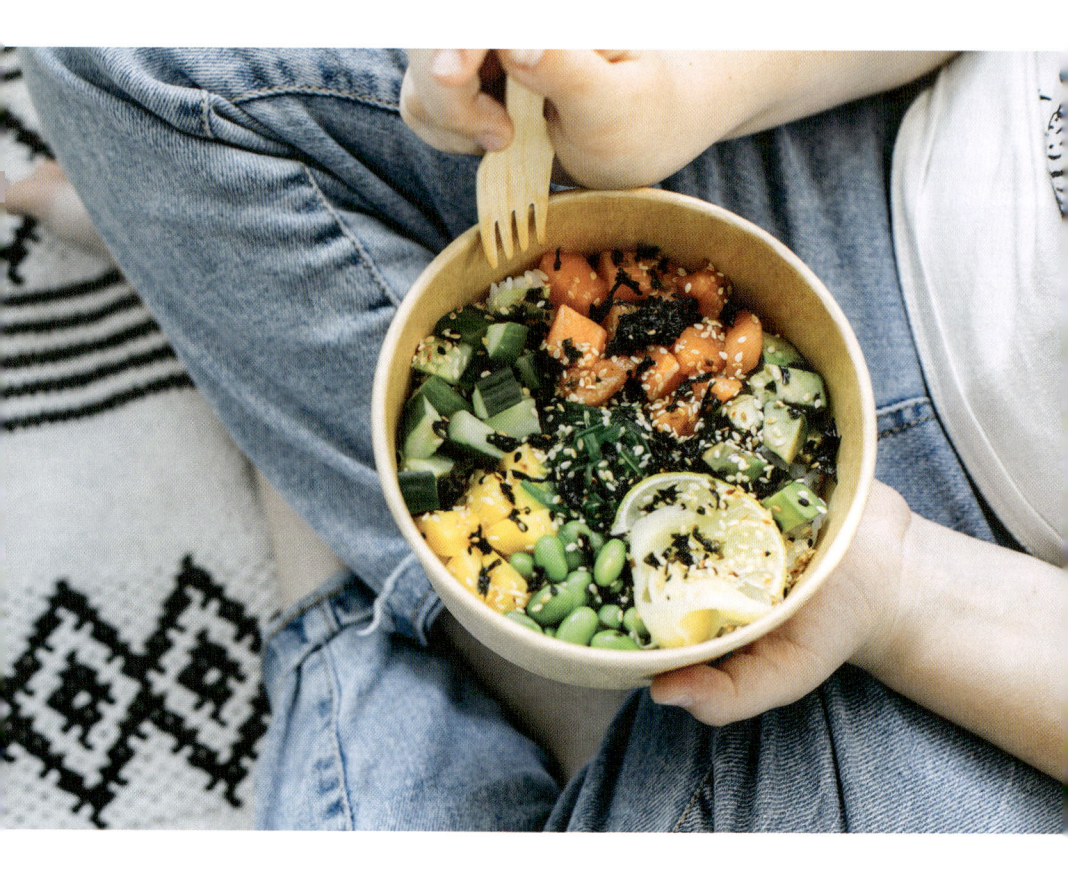

MEAL TIMING

Meal timing is a tricky beast. It can be really useful in certain situations, and other times meaningless or confusing. If it feels overwhelming to try to piece together your nutrition action plan, I recommend saving meal timing for last or skipping it altogether.

Some principles of meal timing:

- Eat at regular intervals.
- Eat approximately the same amount of food at each meal.
- Pay attention to timing your food intake around workouts.

However, meal timing can make a difference in feeling great and well fueled. When you exercise, you are putting a stressor on your body. Your body needs nutrients to recover, rebuild, repair, and make training adaptations such as stronger muscles or a higher cardiovascular capacity. Your body is recovering for 24–48 hours after a workout. This means it really likes to have a steady supply of nutrients to facilitate this recovery.

EAT AT REGULAR INTERVALS

This would look like meals spaced every 3 to 4 hours apart, with snacks in between as needed. Less optimal—or even detrimental—is going for large windows of time without eating. Some research has shown that even within-day energy deficits can cause negative health outcomes.

Regular meals also promote regular digestion and help curb binge eating and overeating. Many people feel out of control with food, or wonder why they feel like they have to eat so many treats at night, but don't realize that this is caused by under-eating throughout the day. If you are overeating at night, it is likely your body asking you for more nutrients. It really could have used those earlier in the day in the form of healthful meals and snacks.

Let's use an example of two cross-country skiers.

	Skier 1	**Skier 2**
Breakfast	Oatmeal, milk, walnuts, berries, eggs	Skip
Snack	Protein bar	Skip
Lunch	Turkey sandwich, smoothie, carrot sticks	Turkey sandwich, smoothie, carrot sticks
Snack	Crackers and cheese	Skip
Dinner	Pasta with chicken and pesto, salad	Pasta with chicken and pesto, salad
Snack	Peanut butter and apple slices	Ice cream, cookies, chips, and popcorn

Do you identify with one or the other? Some signs you may need to eat more regularly include:

- You feel "binge-y" or overeat, especially at the end of the day.
- It is hard to concentrate.
- You feel irritable, shaky, or sleepy in the middle of the day.
- Your workouts feel more difficult than they should.

- You are not seeing training progress and should have experienced some gains by now.
- You are constipated.
- You feel bloated or easily stuffed after you eat (even if it is a small or normal amount of food).
- You feel like you are not recovering well after workouts (sore muscles, headaches, fatigue, injuries).

EAT THE SAME AMOUNT OF FOOD AT EACH MEAL

This looks like utilizing the plate method as shown above. Or eating at least 500–600 calories per meal—you may need more than this depending on your own goals and body. This also means eating a balanced meal that includes all macronutrients and a variety of food groups.

PAY ATTENTION TO TIMING YOUR FOOD INTAKE AROUND WORKOUTS

This means being mindful of your schedule and the structure of the day.

You want to be able to go into a workout well fueled and hydrated to optimize performance and recovery. You also want to feel good during that workout and not bogged down by a huge meal.

Some principles of meal timing around workouts:

Before

If you have 3 to 4 hours before your workout, you likely have time to eat a full meal. This enables you to be fueled, yet digested so the meal doesn't interfere with your workout. Don't be the person that eats a huge burrito and then tries to go climb. It isn't going to go well for your stomach! Also, don't be the person that eats a salad before a 10-mile run. A salad isn't enough carbohydrate to fuel the run, and it's too much fiber to be digested quickly and supply needed energy.

Add a simple carb within 30–60 minutes of your workout, if it's been a few hours since your last meal.

If you only have 30–90 minutes before the workout, opt for at least 30 grams of simple carbs. See the list on page 32 for lots of ideas.

During

Aim for 30–90 grams of carbs per hour (needs vary depending on many factors).

After

Eat a full meal within 2 hours, including at least 30–60 grams of carbs and 20–40 grams of protein. Try to include a variety of food groups and all macronutrients. This may include fish with potato, salad, and milk. Or tofu with rice, vegetables, and a smoothie.

If you are in a situation where you don't have time to eat right away—like you have a long drive to the next restaurant after your hike, or you need to set up camp before it gets too dark—try getting at least a quick snack in. Things like bottled protein shakes, Gatorade, or a granola bar can help the recovery process until you have time for a full meal.

NUTRITION PERIODIZATION

Periodization refers to a method of matching your nutrition to your training cycle. For example, if you are in the offseason and have a very light training load, you would not need as many calories and carbohydrates as when you are on a backpacking trip hiking 10 or more miles per day.

Similarly, if you are building a cardio base by doing a lot of running, hiking, or cycling, you would need more carbohydrate than if you are in a strength-training phase with very little cardio. Periodization is matching your fueling need to your activity level. A well-known sports nutrition researcher, Dr. Asker Jeukendrup, defines nutrition periodization as "a long-term progressive approach designed to improve athletic performance by systematically varying training throughout the year." And "a planned, purposeful, and strategic use of specific nutritional interventions to enhance the adaptations targeted by individual exercise sessions or periodic training plans, or to obtain other effects that will enhance performance longer term."

Another sports nutrition researcher, Dr. Louise Burke, describes matching your fueling needs as "fuel for the work required." If your "work required" is scaling a mountain, that will take more energy than a 60-minute lifting session at the gym. Fuel according to what you are doing!

Periodization can be applied to different time frames. You can think of periodizing as matching your fueling to day-to-day workouts. You can also match it to week-over-week cycles, or entire training blocks throughout the year.

For example, if you are going on a 50-mile bike ride, you will not only eat a lot of carbs during the ride itself, but you would also increase your carbs in the days and weeks leading up to the ride in order to fuel all the training rides.

You also need to eat additional carbs when the ride is done for the next 1 to 2 days to facilitate recovery.

If you are planning out your year, and have a long cycling event in March and a big climbing trip in September, you would eat more carbohydrate during the cardio training block leading up to your big March cycling event, about 7–10 grams/kilogram/day. Your protein would be moderate at 1.2–1.6 grams/kilogram/day.

You then may switch to maintenance mode with fewer carbs. When you begin training in June for the big climbing trip, you start eating a bit more carbs, but climbing doesn't demand as much as cycling. You are aiming for about 3–5 grams/kilogram/day, but perhaps adding in more protein at 1.6–1.8 grams/kilogram/day to match the strength training load.

In this way, you can leverage your nutrition to optimize performance and training adaptations. Periodization doesn't have to be complex—it is simply matching your nutrition needs to the exercise output.

THE WRAP-UP

Meal planning doesn't have to be difficult, but some degree of planning your meals and meal timing can help support your body to adapt to the training load you place on it. It can also support your body while you are adventuring. Regular, consistent meal intake is optimal to help your body train and recover appropriately.

Periodization refers to matching your energy and macronutrient needs to the current training load, training block, or season. A rest period in the winter will demand less nutrients and energy intake than an in-season thru-hike. Matching your nutrient intake to your energy output can help support your body in all phases and seasons.

REFERENCES

Fahrenholtz, I. L., A. Sjödin, D. Benardot, Å. B. Tornberg, S. Skouby, J. Faber, J. K. Sundgot-Borgen, and A. K. Melin. "Within-Day Energy Deficiency and Reproductive Function in Female Endurance Athletes." *Scandinavian Journal of Medicine and Science in Sports* 28, no. 3 (March 2018), 1139–46. doi: 10.1111/sms.13030. Epub 2018 Feb 5. PMID: 29205517.

Germini, F., N. Noronha, V. Borg Debono, B. Abraham Philip, P. Drashti, T. Navarro, A. Keepanasseril, S. Parpia, K. de Wit, and A. Iorio. "Accuracy and Acceptability of Wrist-Wearable Activity-Tracking Devices: Systematic

Review of the Literature." *Journal of Medical Internet Research* 24, no. 1 (January 21, 2022), e30791. doi: 10.2196/30791. PMID: 35060915; PMCID: PMC8817215.

Jeukendrup, A. E. "Carbohydrate and Exercise Performance: The Role of Multiple Transportable Carbohydrates." *Current Opinion in Clinical Nutrition and Metabolic Care* 13, no. 4 (July 2010), 452–57. doi: 10.1097/MCO.0b013e328339de9f. PMID: 20574242.

Jeukendrup, A. E. "Periodized Nutrition for Athletes." *Sports Medicine* 47, suppl. 1 (March 2017), 51–63. doi: 10.1007/s40279-017-0694-2. PMID: 28332115; PMCID: PMC5371625.

Marquet, L. A., C. Hausswirth, O. Molle, J. A. Hawley, L. M. Burke, E. Tiollier, and J. Brisswalter. "Periodization of Carbohydrate Intake: Short-Term Effect on Performance." *Nutrients* 8, no. 12 (November 25, 2016), 755. doi: 10.3390/nu8120755. PMID: 27897989; PMCID: PMC5188410.

Mifflin, M. D., S. T. St Jeor, L. A. Hill, B. J. Scott, S. A. Daugherty, and Y. O. Koh. "A New Predictive Equation for Resting Energy Expenditure in Healthy Individuals." *American Journal of Clinical Nutrition* 51, no. 2 (1990), 241–47. doi: 10.1093/ajcn/51.2.241.

Simpson, C. C., and S. E. Mazzeo. "Calorie Counting and Fitness Tracking Technology: Associations with Eating Disorder Symptomatology." *Eating Behaviors* 26 (August 2017), 89–92. doi: 10.1016/j.eatbeh.2017.02.002. Epub 2017 Feb 9. PMID: 28214452.

Wallen, M. P., S. R. Gomersall, S. E. Keating, U. Wisløff, and J. S. Coombes. "Accuracy of Heart Rate Watches: Implications for Weight Management." *PLoS One* 11, no. 5 (May 27, 2016), e0154420. doi: 10.1371/journal.pone.0154420. PMID: 27232714; PMCID: PMC4883747.

3
SPECIAL NUTRITION SITUATIONS

You're bound to find yourself in different situations as an outdoor athlete. Mother Nature doesn't provide potable water or electricity. There is no fridge, there is no oven. There's just you and your gear.

High altitude, extreme heat or cold, and other unfavorable conditions also demand specialized fueling and hydration to keep your body functioning properly. Staying safe in the elements is more than high-quality gear. It's understanding how to fuel and hydrate.

Consider this story from Ambrea. Her husband is a salty sweater and loses about 2 liters of fluid per hour. While they were gravel biking, he was struggling due to the heat and excessive sweating. He was vomiting and shivering from heat exhaustion. He was cramping so much that they could not finish the ride. He was struggling so much that he had to stash his bike and hike. They flagged down a truck and hitched a ride back into town. He recovered by resting and adding a lot of fluid and sodium from Gatorade, Coke, pickles, and pizza.

How could this have gone differently if he had planned for the extreme heat? It's hard to say, but certainly being aware of how much fluid and sodium you need is a good start. Sometimes Mother Nature wins and the conditions are not safe to exercise in, but usually with a good fueling and hydration plan, you can find success.

There are also all the other scenarios an outdoor athlete may find themselves in, such as living in a van, traveling across time zones, or sustaining an injury. All these situations can be managed with nutrition.

Here's what we will cover in this chapter:

- Altitude
- Heat/humidity
- Cold
- Van life
- Vegan/vegetarian
- Digestive issues
- Youth and adolescent nutrition
- Masters nutrition
- Female athletes
- Para/adaptive athletes
- Traveling nutrition
- Injury/surgery prevention and recovery

This chapter was designed for you to be able to flip to the section that applies to you. It can be a useful reference for years to come for whatever situation you encounter.

This chapter will give you more specific nutrition strategies for many outdoor scenarios, but still supports the overarching goals mentioned in Chapter 1:

- Eat enough to support basic body processes.
- Eat enough to support training and movement (before, during, and after activity).
- Eat a healthful diet made of mostly whole grains, fruits/vegetables, nuts/seeds, dairy products, and lean protein.
- Refuel and rehydrate after workouts to promote recovery.
- Maintain a good relationship with food, body, and sport.

ALTITUDE

INTRODUCTION

Outdoor adventures often take you to a higher altitude than where you may live. Getting altitude sickness on the big trip you've been training for is a

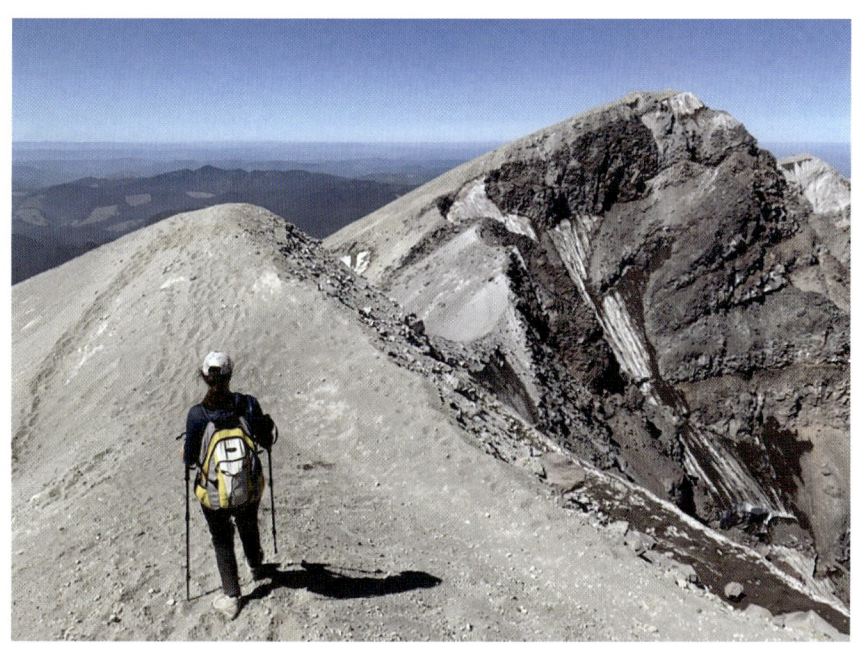

The author on Mount St. Helens

nightmare. Months of planning can fall apart if your body doesn't cooperate at high altitude.

Having a nutrition and hydration plan is key to any high-altitude adventure. If you don't have a strategy, you may find yourself fatigued, injured, or sick.

First, how is *high altitude* defined? It depends on whom you ask, but usually it is around the following:

- Lower altitude: 1,000–2,000 meters (3,280–6,561 feet)
- Moderate altitude: 2,000–3,000 meters (6,561–9,842 feet)
- High altitude: 3,000–5,000 meters (9,842–16,404 feet)
- Extreme altitude: >5,000 meters (>16,404 feet)

HOW ALTITUDE AFFECTS YOUR BODY
- At high altitudes, the air is thinner, meaning the oxygen molecules are spread farther apart than at sea level. This means you may feel a bit short of breath for every inhale. You're simply getting less oxygen per breath than you're used to—especially if you live at a lower altitude and are going up to a high altitude.
- Some stress hormones, such as cortisol and adrenaline, increase. This increases carbohydrate demand in your body.
- Basal metabolic rate is also increased.
- Some people experience a loss of appetite, due to changes in appetite-regulating hormones leptin, cholecystokinin, and ghrelin.
- Respiratory fluid losses are greater. This means for every breath exhaled, you are losing more fluid than you would have at sea level. Which means you need more fluid than normal to stay properly hydrated.
- Urinary losses are greater, which further emphasizes the need for adequate fluids.
- There is a decrease in exercise capacity due to the thin air and lower oxygenation throughout your body, due to decreased cardiac capacity. This may mean you cannot go as fast, or as intense as you could at sea level. Plan for a slower pace and be aware of your daily schedule. Knowing that you may need to cover less ground in a given day can help keep you safe. For instance, if you usually can hike 5 miles in 2 hours, but you are at a high altitude, you may only hike 3 miles in 2 hours. This can alter your schedule if you have to set up camp before

sunset or reach a certain trail marker at a certain time. A slow ascent (600–1,200 meters per day above 2,500 meters) can give your body time to adapt and prevent altitude sickness.
- Sleep may be compromised, which means your recovery may suffer. If you are at high altitude for a number of days and are relying on your body to perform difficult tasks, recovery and sleep are crucial to keep your brain and body functioning optimally.

NUTRITION STRATEGIES

Iron

Since iron is involved with delivering oxygen to tissues in your body (lungs, heart, muscles), it's important to have adequate iron stores.

Get your iron levels checked at least 6–8 weeks before your trip. Make an appointment with your doctor to get a full iron panel. It usually includes serum iron, total iron binding capacity, ferritin stores, and transferrin saturation.

If any deficiencies are detected, your doctor can recommend a correct dose and form of iron to take. It's not a good idea to just take iron supplements on your own, especially if you don't know if you are deficient or anemic. Test, don't guess. If you take iron when you don't need it, you could cause iron overload in your body, known as hemochromatosis.

Food sources of iron that are good to incorporate in your diet include:

- Shellfish
- Spinach
- Lentils
- Beef
- Quinoa
- Turkey
- Tofu
- Dark chocolate
- Fortified breakfast cereal

Note that plant sources of iron are absorbed less efficiently than animal sources. See the vegan/vegetarian section for more information.

Cooking in a cast iron skillet and eating foods with vitamin C help iron absorption as well (citrus foods and berries are common sources of vitamin C).

Calories

Outdoor athletes who spend a lot of time at high altitude sometimes unintentionally lose weight. This can be due to several reasons, including the fact that your body is under stress and uses more calories, you may not have access to as much food as usual, and you are working harder than usual due to your outdoor activities. Appetite is sometimes decreased in higher altitudes, which also makes it difficult to get enough food. Energy expenditure from a few studies of alpinists at high elevation show they use between 3,500 and 5,500 calories daily.

To combat accidental weight loss, try eating high-calorie foods (trail mix, nut butter, fluids with calories, protein bars, chocolate, ghee), adding fat (oils, butter, sauces, gravies) to foods, and packing more food than you think you will need.

Fluids

A good hydration strategy is key to successful high-altitude trips! Your body needs more fluids because not only is it stressed, but the air is usually more arid (less moisture). With each breath, you lose some moisture from your body. Sweating, respiration (breathing), and urinary losses are all greater at high altitude.

There is about a 3 percent decrease in exercise capacity for every 300 meters above 1,500 meters. That can add up to a big difference as you ascend.

Overall blood volume may decrease, which is a bad thing for your exercise performance. With each heartbeat, your body is pumping less blood and less oxygen throughout your body. This can lead to fatigue and failed attempts at summiting, sending, or whatever your goal is.

Always pack more water than you think you need, and/or bring along a water filter if your route has water nearby. Research shows that people are more prone to drink adequate amounts if the water is flavored. Enhance your fluids by using sports drinks or flavored electrolyte powders or tablets.

Electrolytes are also crucial to hydrating properly. You lose sodium, calcium, magnesium, and potassium in sweat. If you're only drinking water and not replacing electrolytes, you're setting yourself up for dehydration or overhydration. See Chapter 1 for more on hydration.

Aim for at least 3–5 liters per day (13–21 8-ounce cups). Don't rely on thirst, as this can be unreliable in extreme conditions. Drink at regular intervals every 20–30 minutes to stay ahead of the hydration game. Watch your urine color—it should be light yellow, like lemonade. If it is too dark (like tea or cola), concentrated, or has a strong odor, you are likely dehydrated. This can take hours or even a full day to recover from.

It may be tempting to skip hydrating because, let's face it, it's a pain to pee in the wilderness. Don't let the inconvenience of urinating stop you from adequately hydrating. A pit stop to relieve yourself is way more convenient than becoming dehydrated or having a medical emergency in the middle of nowhere.

Carbohydrates

Carbs are king when it comes to fueling outdoor adventures. They are the main fuel source for your brain and muscles. At high altitudes, the hormones cortisol and adrenaline kick in. Cortisol is a stress hormone that demands more carbohydrates. In addition, the work you are doing to execute your adventure is also using carbohydrates.

Fuel regularly by eating every 20–30 minutes. Eat a few bites of carbohydrate-rich foods, such as:

- Sports gummies and chews
- Fruit snacks
- Dried fruit
- Fruit leather
- Crackers, chips, pretzels
- Sports drinks with carbs
- Gu or gels
- Gummies, like Swedish Fish or Sour Patch Kids
- Bagels

If your blood sugar drops, you may feel weak, shaky, dizzy, fatigued, or have a headache. Luckily, with some carbohydrates in your body, you can recover from low blood sugar within about 20–30 minutes (a much faster recovery time than dehydration). Take a rest and eat some food. Aim for minimum 30–60 grams of carbs per hour of activity.

You may also want to try beet juice, powder, or shots. There is some evidence that suggests the nitrate in beets (which converts to nitric oxide in your body) may help at high altitudes. Nitric oxide opens blood vessels to allow for more blood flow and oxygenation.

> **LOGISTICS TIPS FOR HIGH-ALTITUDE TRIPS AWAY FROM HOME**
>
> Plan and purchase all food in the nearest town before your excursion. To prevent foodborne illness, avoid drinking local water and ice cubes if you are in a country where clean water may not be reliable—instead, use bottled water or bring a specialized water bottle with a straw filtration system built into it. Avoid raw fruits and vegetables and do not eat from street vendors. Keep animals and restroom areas far away from food storage and prep areas.
>
> If your appetite is low, avoid high-fiber foods (since they are filling but lower in calories) and use fluids with calories, such as juice, milk, protein shakes, sports drinks, and soups. Eat on a schedule—such as one snack every hour, and one meal every 3 hours.
>
> If you are using a guide company, communicate with them beforehand to ensure you understand what food will be provided. Some provide all food or one or two meals daily. Make sure you know what to expect, and plan your food accordingly.

Always bring more fuel, food, and water than you think you will need! You never know when your trip will take longer than planned, weather conditions may change, or someone around you may need some food or fluids. Be prepared for any situation.

While this isn't a nutrition strategy, most scientific literature recommends sleeping at altitude or in altitude tents to acclimatize your body. You may also consider a slow ascent, no more than 500–1,000 meters per day. For example, risk of altitude sickness drops when climbers of Mount Kilimanjaro take more than 7 days and a slow ascent. Diomax (acetazolamide) is a medication that is often used to prevent altitude sickness. Check with your doctor to see if this is appropriate for you. It can cause dehydration, so use caution with this drug.

HEAT

INTRODUCTION

You have probably felt the effects of heat if you go on a hike or ride when you are not used to the hot weather. Most people feel slower and sluggish. Heat and humidity can range from bothersome and uncomfortable to life-threatening and dangerous.

If you have the option of traveling to your destination to acclimatize yourself to the heat, do so about 2 to 3 weeks before your big adventure. You could also consider using a sauna if you have access to one—many gyms and spas have saunas available. Sitting in one on a regular basis can help condition your body to the heat. Use caution and check with your doctor before doing so if you are pregnant, have any heart condition, high blood pressure, or any other condition that would make it unwise to use a sauna.

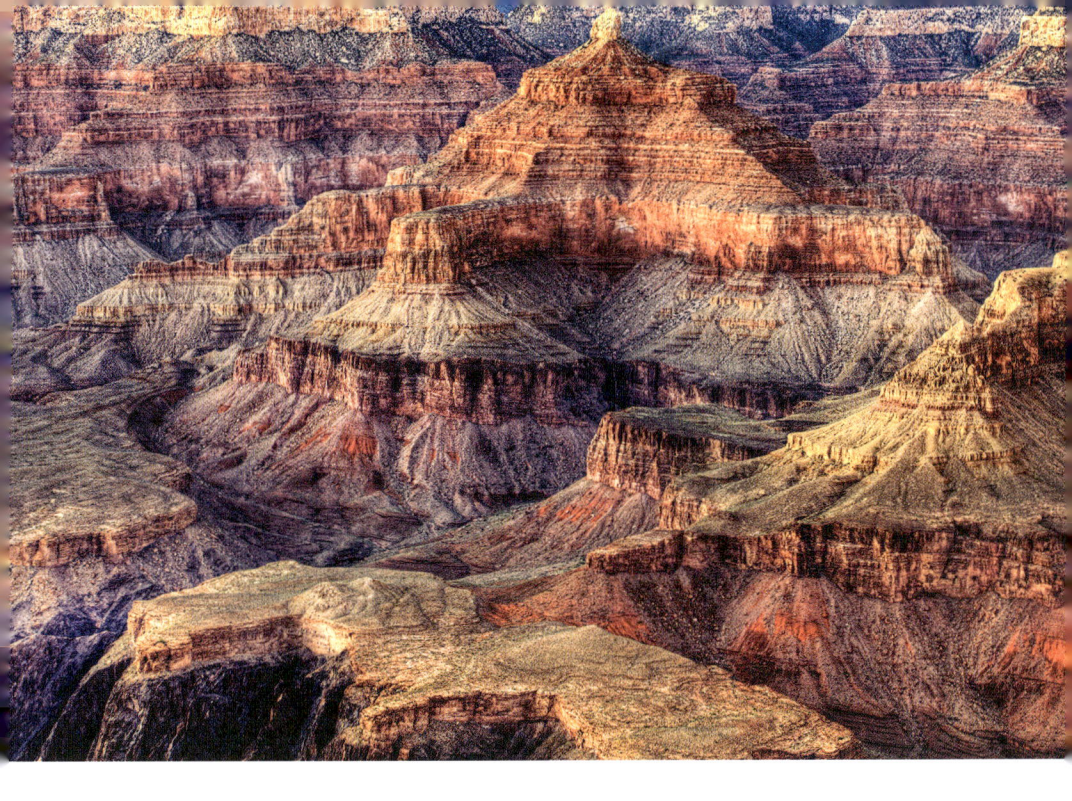

Heat strategies like acclimatization help your body adapt to the heat by decreasing your heart rate while exposed to heat, reducing your skin temperature, and increasing your sweat rate (thereby regulating body temperature more effectively). You may feel and perform better if you've had the chance to acclimatize before embarking on your adventure in the heat.

HOW HEAT AFFECTS YOUR BODY

Hot weather can increase your body temperature, decrease cardiovascular performance, and increase your rate of use of glycogen (that storage form of sugar in your skeletal muscles and liver). This means you may "bonk" or hit the wall sooner than expected unless you fuel properly. In hot weather, fluid losses are greater via sweat. A lower power output and a slower rate of activity overall make it difficult to perform your best. Some people experience a reduced appetite, which can make it challenging to eat enough if you are on an adventure that demands a lot of energy intake to support your activity level. Blood flow to the gut is also reduced, which means some people have a poor appetite or nausea (but the nausea could also be due to depleted glycogen or electrolytes).

NUTRITION STRATEGIES

First, increase your carbohydrate intake in hot weather. Your body needs more carbs to function well. Give it carbs! A minimum suggestion is 30 grams per hour, but you may need much more than this, depending on the duration and intensity of your workout. See Chapter 1 for more details about carbohydrates.

Next, cooling drinks can be really beneficial. Some studies have given subjects a drink with ice or a slushy and found that their body temperature decreased, and it also translated into some performance improvements in very hot weather. This kind of internal cooling can be useful and refreshing. You could also try external cooling, such as dumping water on your head, using a cool, wet towel around your neck, and wearing light layers of clothing that wick sweat away from your skin.

You also need to start your adventure well hydrated. This can be a challenge, especially if you are in the backcountry day after day and may be dehydrated or under-fueled from so many days of exertion. As mentioned before, watch your urine color—make sure it is light yellow—and don't skip drinking just because it is a pain to urinate in the wilderness. Be sure to hydrate well after you are done for the day to set yourself up well for the next day.

If you are not in the wilderness, you may have access to a scale. If you're at home or a hotel for your adventure, you could test your sweat rate and drink accordingly. For more information as to how to test sweat rate, see Chapter 1. Some scientific literature recommends drinking 150 percent of the fluid lost. This means if you lost 1 pound of body weight—which is 16 ounces of fluid—you should then drink 24 ounces to rehydrate.

Even in the heat, there is a possibility of overhydration. This can happen if you are so hot and thirsty you drink too much (especially if you drink only plain water with no electrolytes). You will know if you are overhydrated if you have a sloshy stomach, feel nauseated, or are confused or very slow or feel like you are retaining water. This can be a medical emergency. Avoid drinking too much fluid to avoid the possibility of overhydration.

If you are exercising less than 60 minutes, you can probably drink according to thirst and be safe without a formal hydration plan. For anything over 90 minutes, you can drink 5–6 ml/kg fluid every 2–3 hours before you start

> **HEAT EXHAUSTION VS. HEAT STROKE**
>
> Heat exhaustion and heat stroke are both serious, but heat stroke can be life-threatening and is a medical emergency.
>
> *Heat exhaustion* can happen when your body loses too much water and sodium (the key electrolyte lost in sweat). Symptoms include weakness, fatigue, an increased sweat rate, weak or fast pulse, nausea, vomiting, cold skin, and dizziness. To treat, stop exercising, drink cold fluids with electrolytes, and try to get your body cooled down by taking a cold shower, moving to the shade, and taking off excess clothing. If you can't cool down within 30 minutes or you have vomited, seek medical attention.
>
> *Heat stroke* is when your body temperature is elevated and can no longer regulate itself properly. Symptoms include a rapid, strong pulse, hot dry skin, shortness of breath, slurred speech, and change in consciousness. To treat, call 911 and try to cool the skin with fans/air circulation or a cold compress. Don't drink anything—wait until medical help arrives.

exercising. Heavy sweaters should drink 400 ml every 15 minutes. Specific fluid needs vary widely—use your own experience and judgment. Some people lose 2–3 liters per hour, so know your own sweat rate.

COLD

INTRODUCTION

Your outdoor adventures will likely have you in cold environments. Skiing, ice climbing, snowshoeing, and hiking at high altitudes can all be quite cold. High altitude often produces cooler temperatures than lower elevations. Check back to the altitude section if this applies to your adventure.

In cold environments, the right gear and clothing are important to keep you safe and comfortable, and so is the right nutrition!

HOW COLD AFFECTS THE BODY

Cold temperatures increase fluid losses through respiration. They can also increase fluid losses through sweat if you have so many layers of warm clothing that you perspire. Wet conditions, like a rainstorm, can make clothing wet and make it difficult to maintain body temperature. If you are a swimmer, cold water can suck the heat out of your body—at a rate four times greater than in the air.

Resting metabolic rate can be elevated due to the body's efforts to maintain temperature. Shivering increases metabolic rate and increases the use of carbohydrate/glycogen stores. This means your body will need more calories.

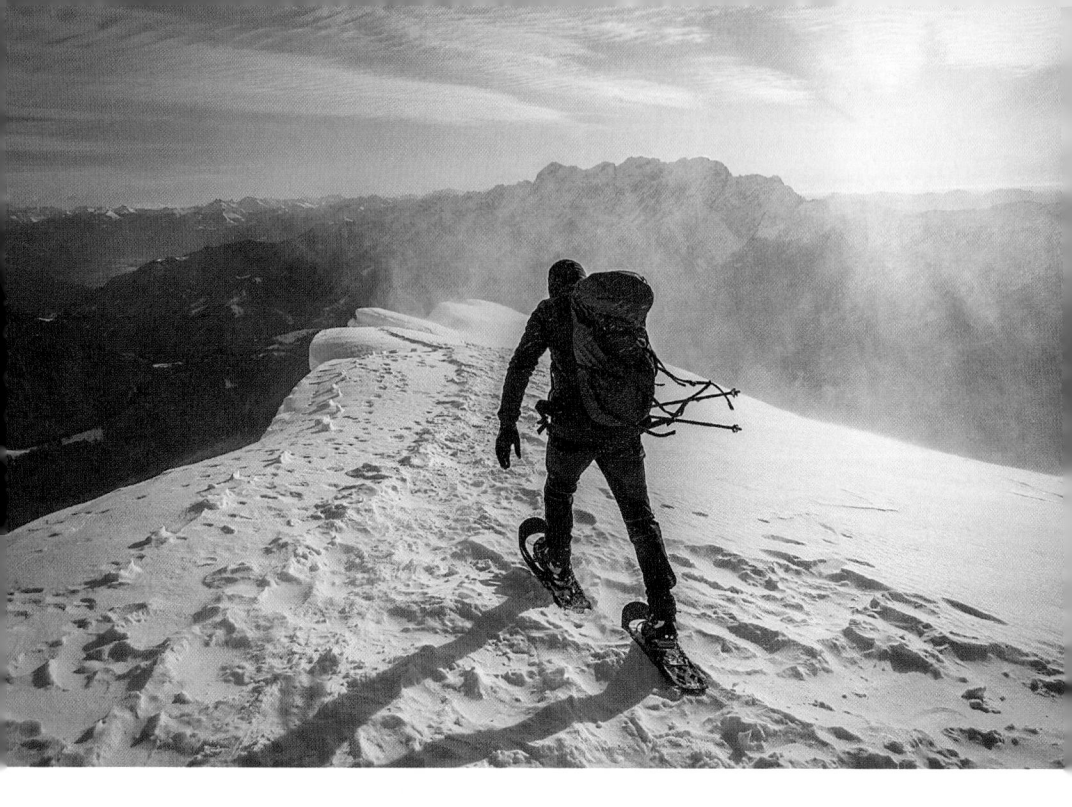

As you may know from experience, cold environments can also seem to limit the range of motion of certain movements. Muscles may feel stiffer, and cold hands cannot perform precise movements as well.

NUTRITION STRATEGIES

Since your metabolic rate is higher in the cold, you will need adequate energy intake. Carbohydrates are also needed in larger quantities than at a normal temperature. Aim for simple carbs if you are doing intense activities, and other carbs and foods at lower intensities. For example, a short, intense ski race lasting a couple of minutes demands simple carbs. A long, slow snowshoe hike that lasts all day can use a mix of simple carbs and more complex foods such as trail mix or jerky.

Calorie-dense foods that don't freeze easily are necessary for some outdoor adventures. Try sports gels, bread, dried fruit, chocolate, honey, puree pouches, granola, dehydrated or freeze-dried meals, sports drinks, milk powder, gummy bears, lentil pouches, cheese, sausages, trail mix, and canned or pouches of tuna. Depending on the conditions, some of these may freeze, but many are good options that don't require cooking, and may not even need glove removal to eat (depending on how they are packaged).

Try opening packaging beforehand if possible, so you don't have to deal with that with gloves on. Also, keeping a rotation of snacks in a warmer inside pocket of your jacket or pants can allow them to thaw before you eat.

If you are able to cook, try adding pasta, rice, quinoa, polenta, instant potatoes, oats, ramen, and instant soup to your menus.

Hot drinks can help raise body temperature. Things like soup, tea, coffee, ramen, and hot chocolate can feel wonderful on a chilly day.

Fluids are a challenge in the cold, especially if they freeze! Depending on your activity, you may be able to carry fluids with you or you may melt snow for water. Even though fluids are a logistical challenge, they are crucial to ensure you stay well hydrated. You may not feel thirsty in cold weather, but you still need to drink. Aim for at least 8 ounces per hour. You may need more if you are in extreme conditions or doing very intense work. Try to avoid bladder-and-hose systems where the hose is very long and could freeze if the temperatures are cold enough.

VAN AND RV LIFE

The dirtbag lifestyle can bring you to some amazing places but also brings challenges with cooking and food storage.

Before embarking on a van journey, plan ahead to cover all the logistics. Some vehicles are fully equipped with fridges, stoves, and cookware. Others are bare bones with a cooler and a camp stove that can only be used outside. Know your vehicle and its features.

Be sure to understand and implement safe cooking practices. Do not use the same cutting board, knife, or utensils for raw meat and other foods. Sanitize your hands after touching raw meat or eggs. Cook meat thoroughly. Store perishable foods at 40 degrees or below. Do not use cooking fuel while indoors.

It's also tempting to skip hydrating adequately if you don't have access to a toilet. Drink regularly to stay hydrated while in the wilderness. You can watch your urine color—it should be light yellow.

Pack non-perishable items and always have these staples on hand. When you get to the nearest town, you can stock up with fresher items if you have the storage capabilities.

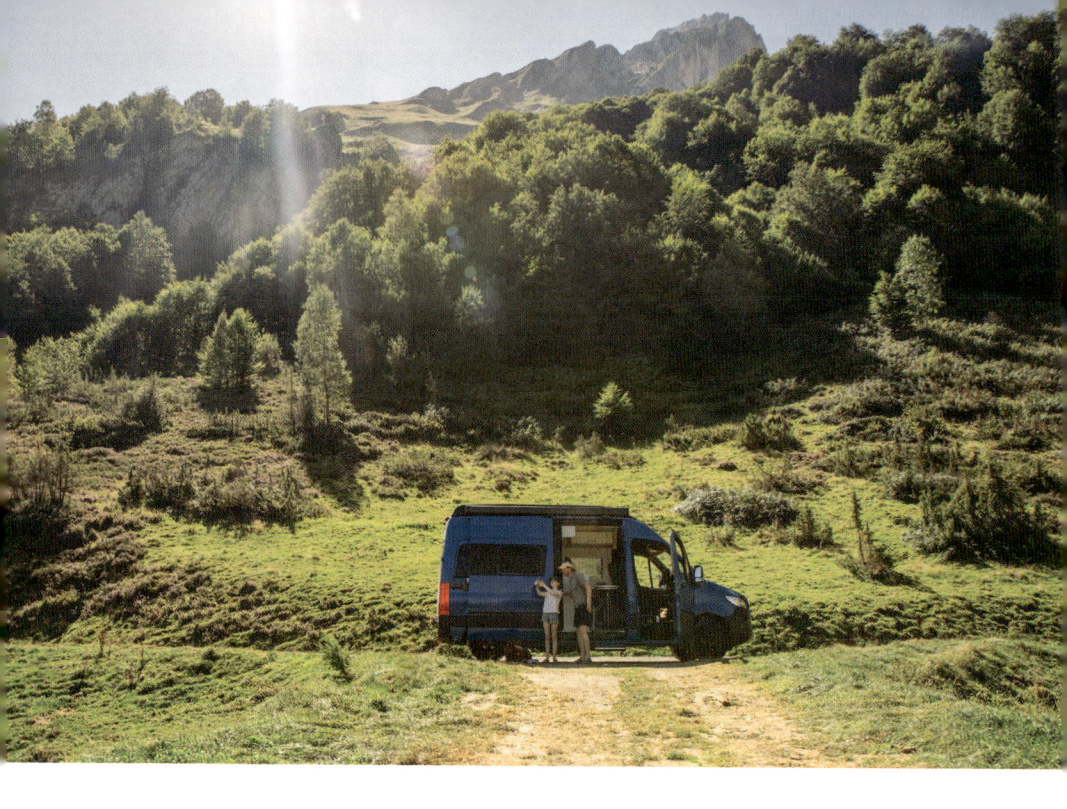

KEY ESSENTIALS

Pot	Cutting board
Pan	Knife
Dish soap	Towel
Dish scrub pad	Fuel
Whisk	Portable sink (if the van or RV does not have one)
Spatula	Plates/cups/bowls/utensils
Cooking spoon	Can opener
Rubber spatula	Storage containers for leftovers
Measuring cups	Cooking thermometer
Measuring spoons	Portable stove

USEFUL OPTIONAL ITEMS

Electric kettle
Small rice cooker
Hot plate
French press or coffee maker
JetBoil or similar system

SHELF-STABLE INGREDIENTS

Oatmeal
Pancake mix
Jarred pasta sauce
Pasta
Ramen
Rice
Quinoa
Shelf-stable protein (canned meats, canned beans, pouch tuna or salmon, pouch pre-cooked lentils, shelf-stable milk or plant milks)
Protein powder or shake mix
Sports drink powder
Nuts/trail mix
Jerky
Eggs or egg powder
Cheese or freeze-dried cheese
Soup (canned or dehydrated)
Peanut butter
Coffee and tea
Protein and granola bars
Condiments (spices, mustard, dressings, honey, ketchup, jam packets)
Dry cereal and granola
Olive oil
Dehydrated/freeze-dried meals and MREs
Boxed drinks (water, milk, juice)
Applesauce or fruit puree pouches

FRESH/PERISHABLE INGREDIENTS

Easy vegetables (bagged salad, baby carrots, cherry tomatoes, small bell peppers, tiny cucumbers, olives, celery, canned or frozen veggies)
Easy fruit (berries, apples, oranges, bananas, grapes, canned or frozen fruit)
Hummus
Yogurt
Cottage cheese

Meat
Tofu
Bread/bagels/tortillas
Eggs
Cheese
Jam

EASY MEAL IDEAS

Pasta + sauce + salad + chicken
Egg + bagel + salmon + fruit
Quesadillas + chicken + salad
Oatmeal + berries + eggs
Salad + tofu cubes + veggies
Stir fry tofu + veggies + rice
PB & J + apple slices + yogurt
Yogurt + granola + berries

With the right planning, your van trip (or complete van life!) can be a well-fueled success.

VEGAN AND VEGETARIAN DIETS

For some reason, the vegan and vegetarian world is often charged with emotion. Whether you are vegan or vegetarian for environmental reasons, moral, ethical, or religious reasons, or anything else, this section is meant to help support you in that choice. It's important to carefully plan your diet to avoid nutrient deficiencies and optimize your nutrition and fueling.

It is also important to assess whether this dietary choice works for you. Some people can live this dietary pattern quite easily—they do not feel restricted and do not feel like their health is compromised. Others try to go vegan or vegetarian and find themselves tired, stressed, anxious about food, or the diet is masking disordered eating (see Chapter 6 for more on this).

Before starting this diet, reflect on the reasons for doing so, and make sure you fully understand the complex considerations. If you read a book, heard a podcast, or saw a documentary about veganism and are convinced that is the way to go, know that these are usually not sources of valid nutrition information.

Following a vegan or vegetarian diet can be a challenge, as there are obvious dietary restrictions. It is hard to get a wide variety of nutrients whenever there is any type of restriction, especially if nutrient access is limited as an outdoor athlete because you are on a mountaintop, deep in a forest, or in the middle of a body of water. Following a strict diet can also lead to a disrupted relationship with food, and increased anxiety and stress around food.

However, vegans and vegetarians can adopt this lifestyle with some careful planning. Many enjoy living a vegan or vegetarian life with no problems as an outdoor athlete.

NUTRIENT CONSIDERATIONS

Fiber

Because you are eating a lot (or only) plant foods, many vegans and vegetarians naturally get more fiber in their diet than omnivores. This is usually beneficial and health-promoting. A high-fiber diet reduces the risk of chronic disease, helps regulate digestion, and helps manage blood sugar.

The downside is that some people struggle to tolerate so much fiber. They may feel bloated, gassy, or even have cramping or diarrhea. Constipation can result if the fiber intake is not matched with adequate fluid intake.

Another potential downside is that fiber makes people feel full. While this sounds good on the surface, if a high-fiber meal interferes with your ability to ingest enough calories to support your activity levels, you could be at risk for nutrient deficiencies and relative energy deficiency in sport (REDs). See Chapter 6 for more details on this condition.

The take-home message is that, while fiber is an important part of a healthful diet, pay attention to how it affects *you*. If you notice gastrointestinal issues or symptoms of REDs, consider reducing fiber intake or talk with a dietitian.

Iron

This key nutrient is a challenge for vegans and vegetarians. Because plant sources of iron are not as well absorbed as animal sources, some may need to supplement with iron pills. In addition, many nutrients in plants—such as calcium in green leafy vegetables, or zinc in whole grains—compete with iron absorption. Phytates, a compound found in some legumes, nuts, and soy, also can limit absorption by binding to the iron in your body. The recommended daily iron intake is higher for vegans and vegetarians for this reason: 33 milligrams daily. Menstruating people, distance runners, and other endurance athletes also have higher iron needs due to greater losses.

Why are you worried about iron as an outdoor athlete? Because iron helps red blood cells transport oxygen into the cells, which is a part of cell metabolism. If you are low on iron, you could feel more fatigued, easily winded, irritable, have headaches, feel lightheaded, and have trouble regulating body temperature. It's important to keep adequate iron status in your body. If you think you may be deficient or anemic, check with your doctor.

If you need to supplement with iron, pairing it with vitamin C helps with absorption. Try your iron supplement with some orange juice or berries. Iron supplements also sometimes cause constipation. You can mitigate this by taking your supplement with a meal, or taking it every other day. Check with your doctor for the right dose and form of iron supplement that is most appropriate.

Vitamin D

The "sunshine vitamin" may be produced in your body if you have enough exposure to sunlight, but this can be a challenge. Dark skin, sunscreen, protective clothing, training indoors, and living at northern or southern latitudes over 32 degrees is a recipe for vitamin D deficiency. Even if you spend a lot of time outdoors, you may still be deficient.

This is a supplement worth considering for many people. Check with your doctor to get your vitamin D status measured (this is usually a standard blood draw) to see if you need to supplement. Food sources are scarce but include fortified milk, yogurt, breakfast cereal, orange juice, and egg yolks.

Calcium

This mineral is usually not difficult for vegetarians to consume if they include dairy in their diet. Vegans, however, may have a harder time. Plant sources are not as bioavailable. A calcium supplement may be necessary, but always check with your doctor first. Vegetarian-friendly sources of calcium include calcium-set tofu, calcium-fortified orange juice, almonds, legumes, calcium-fortified plant milks, kale, collard greens, and texturized vegetable protein. Making sure you are getting enough vitamin D is also important since calcium absorption in the body is reduced if vitamin D status is deficient.

Vitamin B12

Vegans must pay attention to this crucial vitamin. Since it is only found in animal products, vegans must supplement with vitamin B12. This is vital to avoid deficiency. Vegetarians can get B12 from dairy products and eggs, but still should get periodic testing to ensure their vitamin B12 levels are adequate to avoid anemia or long-term nerve damage.

Zinc

Like many other nutrients, zinc is more poorly absorbed from plant sources as compared to animal sources. Zinc absorption is hampered by phytic acid—found in many plant sources. Legumes and whole grains are good sources of zinc. Soaking or sprouting these foods can enhance absorption. Other good sources are seeds, nuts, fortified breakfast cereal, hard cheese, and soy products.

Omega-3 Fatty Acids

These are a category of fat that can be anti-inflammatory and have positive health outcomes, especially in relation to cardiovascular disease. There is also some research on using this type of fatty acids for concussion recovery. For more on injury recovery, see page 77.

Omega-3 fatty acids are found in egg yolks if the chickens are given a special feed. They are also in fish such as salmon, oysters, sardines, and mackerel. Since fish is off-limits for vegans and vegetarians, fortunately, there are some plant sources. Walnuts, chia seeds, soybeans, and flax and hemp seeds and oils all contain omega-3 fatty acids. However, these are not utilized in the body as efficiently as the animal sources. If you want to take a supplement, you can use algal oil. Always check with your doctor before taking any supplements.

Creatine

This is found in meat, so vegans and vegetarians cannot get this from their diet. This is not an essential nutrient, and your body makes some creatine. However, vegans and vegetarians have been found in some studies to have lower stores than omnivores. Vegans and vegetarians who supplement with creatine may find increased power, longer time to fatigue, and increased lean muscle mass, since creatine can have beneficial effects on sports performance. Check with your doctor before supplementing, especially if you have a kidney disease or history of kidney problems. For more about creatine, see Chapter 4.

Protein

You may have heard that vegans and vegetarians cannot get enough protein in their diet. This is not true. As long as the diet is planned carefully, it is totally possible for a vegetarian and, yes, even a vegan, to get enough protein. Some research suggests that vegans and vegetarians may need about 10 percent more protein than omnivores. This is because plant proteins are less easily utilized in the body than animal proteins. It is also more difficult to digest plant proteins due to the fiber content.

To mitigate this problem, be mindful of how much protein you need. Try to get your protein from a variety of plant sources. Soy products like tofu and tempeh are great sources. You can also use protein powders (look for a blend, not just a single source), hemp, peas, lentils, legumes, quinoa, and whole grains, and some meat and "milk" substitutes can be good sources of protein as well. Vegetarians can also include eggs and dairy products, which are a readily bioavailable source of complete protein.

TROUBLESHOOTING DIGESTIVE ISSUES

INTRODUCTION

No one wants diarrhea in the backcountry. Bloating, constipation, nausea, abdominal cramping, or loose stool can really put a damper on any outdoor adventure.

Digestive issues can range from mildly annoying to severe, life-threatening symptoms. Some issues are transient, while others are rooted in disease. If you have chronic digestive issues, it's wise to get a full workup by a gastroenterologist to determine if you have any serious conditions such as allergies, celiac disease, Crohn's disease, or ulcerative colitis.

Barring any serious conditions, this section will be helpful to manage symptoms that may be dependent on the foods you eat. We will focus on strategies to manipulate food and fluid intake to help with symptoms. It is out of the scope of this chapter to talk about medical nutrition therapy for digestive symptoms caused by an underlying condition, including intolerances and allergies.

NUTRITION STRATEGIES

You may need to play detective to figure out the root cause of your digestive issues. Don't do this alone. A registered dietitian is an invaluable resource. The nutrition strategy you use depends on the situation and the symptoms.

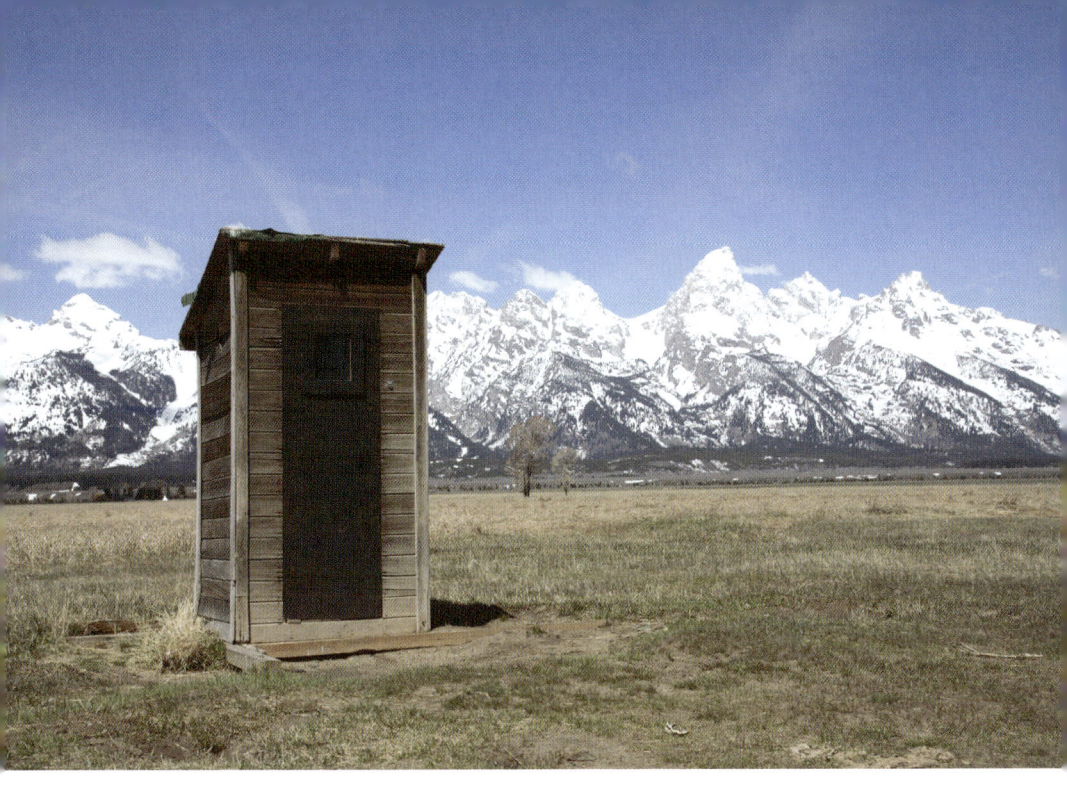

Stomach Upset or Heartburn

Consider avoiding things that may exacerbate indigestion, such as:

- Alcohol
- Caffeine
- Ibuprofen
- Aspirin
- Spicy foods
- Greasy, fried, or fatty foods
- Peppermint
- Acidic foods
- Sugar alcohols (found in many protein bars)

Eat at regular intervals in moderate portion sizes. This is usually better tolerated than skipping a meal and eating very large portions later on.

Nausea/Vomiting

This could be caused by many things, including:

- Low blood sugar
- Overhydration
- Dehydration
- Food poisoning

3 / SPECIAL NUTRITION SITUATIONS

- Anxiety/nervousness (common at a competition)
- Hyperosmolar solutions
- Too much food too close to your exercise

Treat the nausea based on the cause. If it's *low blood sugar*, eat enough carbohydrates and overall food at regular intervals, no more than 4 hours apart. If you are at a high altitude or working at a high intensity, you will need carbs more often—at least every hour.

You need time to recover from *overhydration*. Stop drinking so much if your stomach is sloshy, your urine is clear, you are experiencing frequent urination, or your feet are swollen. This could be a medical emergency, especially if coupled with confusion. Seek medical help immediately. One way to avoid overhydration is to add electrolytes with fluids and know your fluid needs and sweat rate.

You also need time to recover from *dehydration*—up to 24 hours or more. This could also be a medical emergency depending on the severity. Drink fluids with electrolytes. This helps get the fluid into the right spaces in the body, and helps the body retain the fluid rather than producing more urine. Stop exercising and find a safe place to rest, or if possible, seek medical help or go home/back to civilization.

Food poisoning is the outdoor athlete's worst nightmare. It will need to run its course, but you may need medical attention if you become dehydrated from diarrhea or vomiting. Electrolyte fluid solutions can help, as well as antibiotics in some cases. Be sure to practice good food safety, such as cooking food thoroughly and washing/sanitizing hands before cooking and eating.

Anxiety can make any stomach upset if you are really worked up about what you are about to do! Whether it's a via ferrata, surf competition, a high-risk hike, or anything else, nerves can cause nausea or decreased appetite. They can also make stools loose and cause increased urination. Manage this by only eating bland foods, such as chicken, rice, crackers, bread, and fruit or whatever you know you can tolerate. Never eat anything new on competition day (or the few days leading up to it). If you suffer from repeat bouts of nausea due to nerves, try deep breathing or consider seeing a sports psychologist.

Hyperosmolar solution means what you are drinking is more concentrated than blood. This means the intestine has trouble absorbing everything at once. If this is happening, it may feel like gurgling, cramping, diarrhea, nausea, or a sloshy stomach.

This may occur when you are trying to fuel yourself properly and adequately (good job!). But if you are aiming for a large amount of carbs per hour—like 60–90 grams or more—you could have stomach upset if the carbs are only one source. Your intestine has a limited number of receptors to help absorb the carbohydrate. It can only absorb so much glucose at one time. The way to get around this is to eat carbs from multiple sources, such as glucose and fructose. You can also avoid highly concentrated beverages and sports drinks. You can also train your gut to tolerate higher amounts of carbs over a series of months during a normal training block.

Too much food probably doesn't need much explaining. If you have ever tried sprinting after eating a heavy meal, you know what this feels like. If you're prone to nausea and vomiting, eat no less than 2 hours before your event. If you have to eat close to or during the event, make sure it is simple, well-tolerated carbs. Avoid high-fat, high-protein, and high-fiber foods.

Diarrhea

Nothing can ruin a trip like diarrhea can. There are many causes of diarrhea. Like other gastrointestinal issues, you may have to do a bit of detective work or look at your activities in context to determine what is causing the diarrhea. Some common causes are discussed below.

Travelers' diarrhea/food poisoning: Usually occurring due to contamination, this may resolve on its own. Some people may opt to use antibiotics to treat the infection. It could also be caused by general stomach upset from eating unfamiliar food. Dehydration is the main concern here. Be sure to stay hydrated and use oral rehydration solutions if they are available. Seek medical attention if it is severe or you become dehydrated. Prevent travelers' diarrhea by only using bottled water, avoiding ice made with tap water, brushing your teeth with bottled water, avoiding fresh fruits and vegetables, and avoiding food from street vendors or restaurants with poor sanitation. This can be a concern in some countries.

Too much carbohydrate in sports drinks or gels. This may happen if you are trying to nail your fueling, but use a single carbohydrate source or too much carbohydrate at once. Some sports drink powders have a very high concentration of carbohydrate. This is not tolerated well by some people, especially if it is coupled with hot weather or a very intense workout. To avoid this, make sure you test your own limits by using the gel or drink in practice settings before you use it for an important or remote event.

Sodium is also important to replenish if you lose a lot in your sweat. This is because sodium helps absorb carbohydrate in food, gels, and sports drinks. Adding sodium sometimes solves the diarrhea problem.

Best practice includes always testing out the food and drink during training sessions, and having both plain water and a sports drink available. This way, you can switch to plain water for hydration if you notice that the sports drink is causing gastrointestinal issues.

Too much fiber: Normally fiber is a good thing. Adequate fiber in your diet helps with regular bowel movements, contributes to a healthy gut microbiome, helps manage blood sugar regulations, and reduces the risk of chronic disease. However, too much fiber too close to (or during) an activity may exacerbate indigestion. Too much fiber eaten all at once—for example, a large smoothie with fruit, spinach, and chia seeds—can also generate loose stools. Opt for simple carbohydrates if you struggle to handle fiber while exercising. See Chapter 1 for a list of ideas.

Menstrual cycle phase: Some people who menstruate notice loose stools in the week before (and/or the week of) their period. This is common and not concerning. But it could be disruptive if you are in the great outdoors and don't want to experience this symptom. Try to stay hydrated, eat fiber-containing foods if you tolerate them, and avoid foods with a natural laxative effect, such as coffee, fruit juice, bran, and prunes.

With these troubleshooting tips, your next adventure will hopefully involve fewer blue bags and poop shovels, and a little more enjoyment of the great outdoors.

YOUTH AND ADOLESCENT NUTRITION

Kids are not tiny adults. They have different nutrition needs and even metabolize nutrients a bit differently than adults. While adults rely on carbohydrates for enhanced sports performance, younger children metabolize fat more readily. They also sweat less than adults and manage their body temperature regulation by dry heat dissipation (as opposed to evaporative cooling in adults).

Children are also growing. While this may sound obvious, it's important to take this into account. Children may need more food during growth spurts, then eat less food for a time. If they are coming along on an outdoor adventure, they can usually just eat what you eat. However, when looking at the big picture, they need medical monitoring to make sure they are growing correctly.

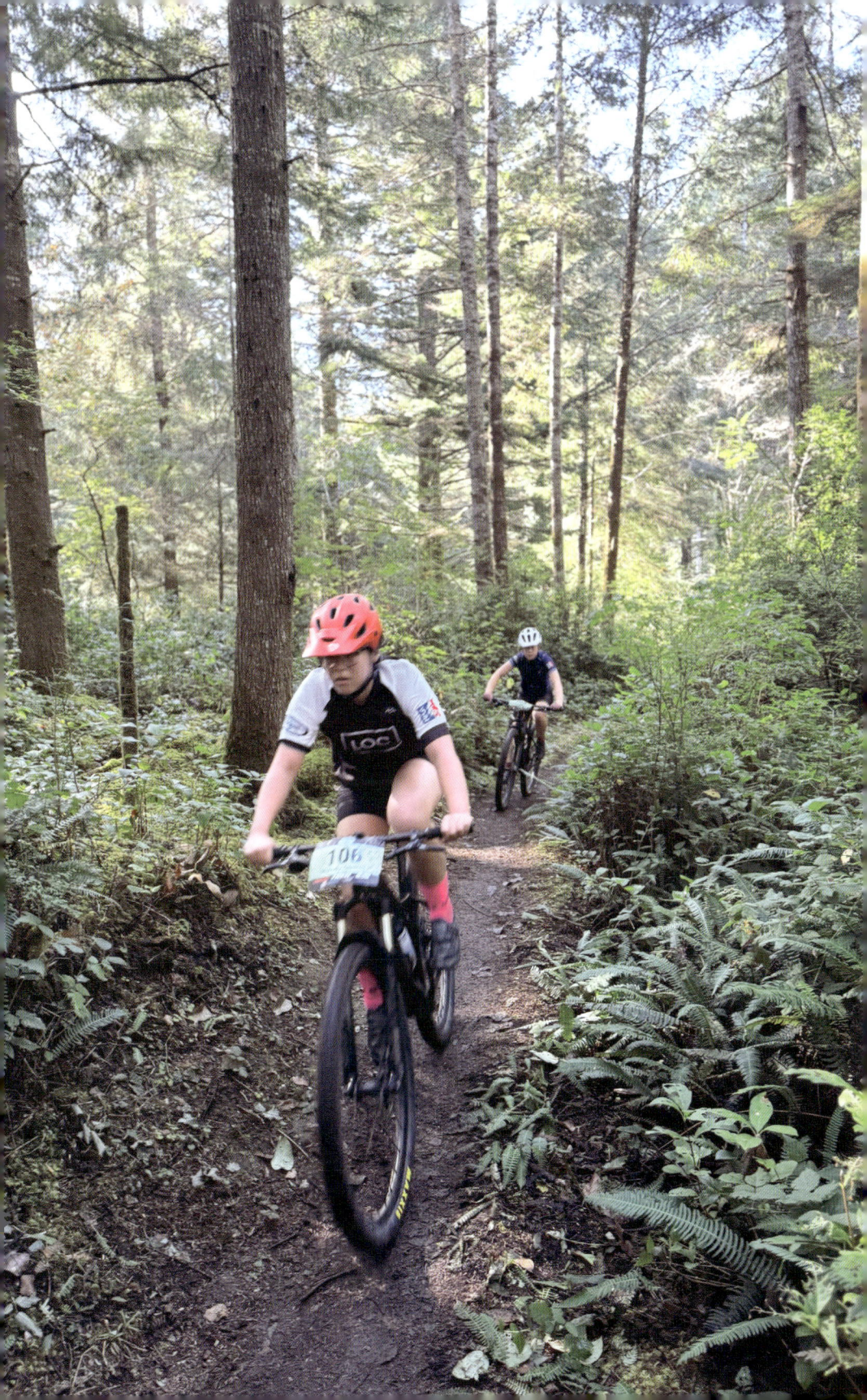

Puberty is a crucial time in a child's life. Until they are in their early 20s, kids are building up bone density and brain volume. They only get one shot at this. If they are underfed, their brain development and bone density may suffer.

Underfeeding usually happens inadvertently. A parent may not realize how much food a kid actually needs, especially a really active kid. Some children are on sports teams, some also have physical education during school, and some play after school outside or have household chores that impose a physical workload. It's important to make sure a kid is getting all the food they need for whatever activity they are doing, in addition to fueling growth and development.

Females can gain 40–50 pounds during puberty and grow 10 inches. Males can gain 50–60 pounds and grow 12 inches or more. It's important to help kids maintain perspective and a positive body image during this time. It can be distressing for some kids to have their body change so much.

Kids participating in weight-class or gravitational sports like climbing, ski jumping, gymnastics, wrestling, and rowing sometimes struggle the most. Their tiny, nimble body that could perform a flip so easily now feels heavier, longer, and awkward. Parents and coaches can help them develop skills, strength, power, and endurance to help them succeed without focusing on their body type. Objectifying a child's body or complimenting them on their small stature can be a recipe for body image disturbances and disordered eating.

Caregivers should take their child to the pediatrician at least on an annual basis for a well-child checkup. There, the pediatrician will measure height and weight to make sure the child is growing properly. These checkups can be invaluable for identifying problems such as poor growth, disordered eating, or nutrient deficiencies.

When participating in outdoor adventures with kids, similar adult fueling principles apply. Regularly fuel and hydrate, bring extra water and snacks, and pay attention to body sensations such as fatigue, temperature regulation, and digestion.

The closer an adolescent is to adulthood, the more their body will function like an adult. A 9-year-old will have different needs than a 16-year-old.

In high heat, for kids ages 9 to 12, aim for about 4 to 8 ounces of fluid every 20 minutes. Aim for 33–50 ounces per hour for kids ages 13–18 years old. Sports drinks are not necessary, but also don't need to be avoided. They can be useful if it helps the kid drink more frequently (due to the flavoring) or if they need some fuel in the form of carbohydrate in the sports drink.

Sports drinks do not need to be used outside of exercise, except in cases of recovery from a very strenuous workout. Children who consume sports drinks all day long (instead of water) are getting additional sodium and sugar that their bodies do not need.

Finally, kids should not use performance-enhancing supplements such as pre-workout blends or creatine. A food-first approach is better for kids, as these supplements are not well researched in an adolescent population. For more on supplements, see Chapter 4.

MASTERS NUTRITION

When I say "masters" I am not talking about skill level. I am talking about age. That's right, if you are older, you are a masters athlete. How old is "older"? It depends on whom you ask, but it is usually around 40 years old. Yes, 40 is not that old. But this marks the age when bodies start changing again. (The term "masters" is also commonly used to refer to participating in formal organizations and competing within age groups. But for this section, it will refer to athletes age 40 and older.)

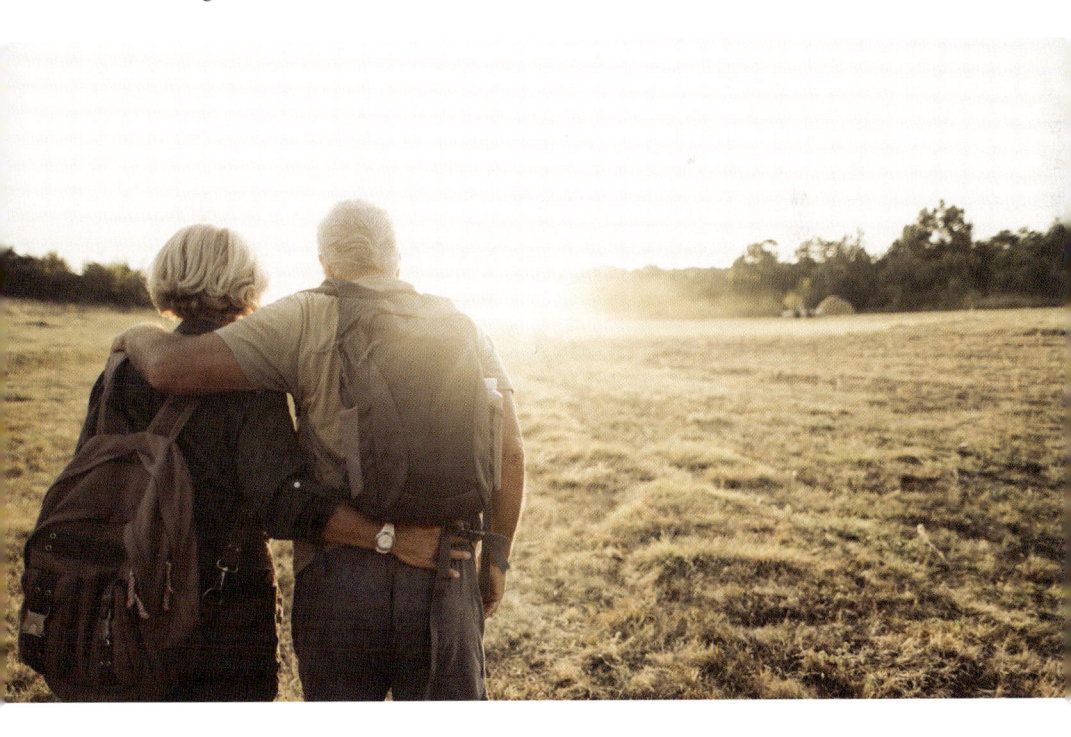

Staying active as you age can be the best thing you can do for overall health. It helps preserve mobility, reduces the risk of cardiovascular disease and diabetes, and helps preserve lean mass as you age.

Physiological differences in masters athletes may include:

- Decreased maximum oxygen uptake capacity (VO$_2$ max)
- Decreased muscle mass and strength
- Increased body fat
- Decreased bone density
- Decreased energy needs (usually beyond age 60)
- Decreased thirst sensations
- Decreased nutrient absorption (past age 60, especially vitamin B12 and iron)

Nutrition strategies include:

- Match carbohydrate needs to training load (more training = more carbohydrate)
- Increase protein intake, to around 35–40 grams per meal
- Monitor fluid intake, sweat rate, and urine color to ensure proper hydration
- Supplement with calcium and vitamin D if indicated to preserve bone health (check with your doctor first)
- Personalize a hydration plan if your thirst sensations have decreased due to age or medication

For specific outdoor adventure fueling, you can follow the general guidelines found throughout this book. Older athletes don't necessarily need different strategies unless they have special circumstances such as reduced kidney function or heart function. Always check with your doctor to make sure you have the correct information for your particular situation.

You can continue to enjoy outdoor activities no matter your age.

FEMALE ATHLETES

NOTE: For the purpose of this section, "female" will refer to cisgender females. Female assigned-at-birth who are trans or nonbinary may find some of this section useful, especially if they are menstruating. The sports performance implications from hormones and other medical treatments for transgender persons are not well known and have limited research. Use your own personal experience and seek appropriate professional guidance for your situation if you have questions about your own physiology and nutrition needs.

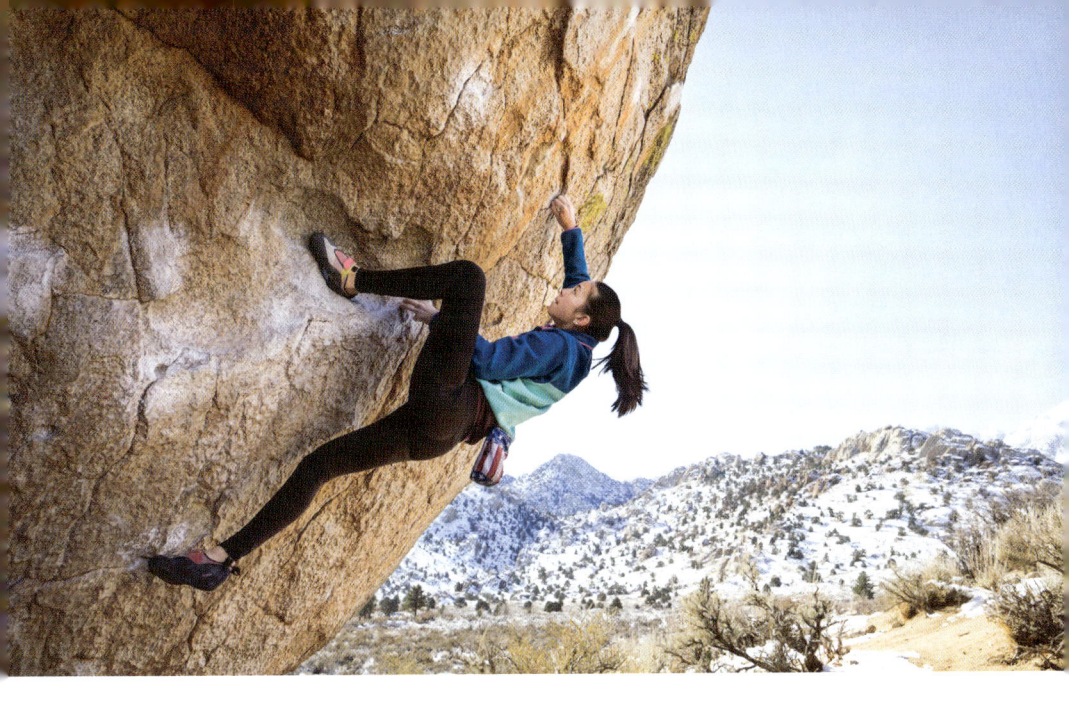

There are whole books dedicated to nutrition and training for females. While it's true that the majority of sports nutrition research has been conducted in males, it's also true that females are not a different species! Females and males have different biology, but many sports nutrition principles apply to all genders.

You may have heard that female outdoor athletes need to train and eat a certain way to match their menstrual cycle. While there are differences in physiology from phase to phase within the menstrual cycle, the differences are not profound enough to warrant much attention to changing the training style or your nutrition.

Recent studies show there are conflicting data as to whether training and nutrition should be altered to match phases. They also conclude that most of the data suggest there is no need to do anything special, as the effect on performance during different phases is trivial.

This is good news for menstruating individuals, as this means you don't have to overthink your training or nutrition. In general, the best guidance is to match your training and nutrition to how your own body is feeling.

For example, if you personally feel like you have low energy, bloating, gastrointestinal issues, or cramps near and during your period, you probably don't feel much like training at a high intensity that day. You could simply alter your plans if possible to include a lighter workload for the day. If you feel energized, regardless of what menstrual phase you are in, you could do a harder workout, go longer, faster, or farther than usual.

If you notice cravings before your cycle, this may be due to blood sugar fluctuations. Your body needs additional energy to make a period happen, which is why some females need an additional 200–500 calories before their period starts. Increased energy and carbohydrate needs could be the cause of cravings. In this case, it may be appropriate to eat more and exercise less, just for a day or two, depending on how your body is feeling. You could also bring more carbohydrate snacks with you on your adventure, to make sure you are fueling enough to meet your body's demands.

Eating adequate protein is also important to help maintain and build lean muscle mass. Most females likely need around 1.4–2.2 grams/kilogram/day. Having protein at each meal and snack will help you reach this goal.

Here is some information to help you understand more about menstrual cycle phases and their performance implications.

The menstrual cycle is divided into two main phases. The follicular phase is roughly day 1 (the first day of your period) through day 15. The luteal phase is roughly day 16–28. These phases are subdivided into smaller phases based on hormonal fluctuations.

Day	Phase	Hormones
1–5	Early follicular	Low estrogen Low progesterone
6–12	Late follicular	High estrogen Low progesterone
13–15	Ovulation	High estrogen Low progesterone
16–19	Early luteal	High estrogen Low progesterone
20–23	Mid luteal	High estrogen High progesterone
24–28	Late luteal	Estrogen and progesterone decline

The hormone estrogen plays a number of roles in regard to exercise performance: It has an anabolic effect (meaning it aids in building muscle tissue), it can regulate substrate metabolism (which can help the cells with utilizing glycogen), and it has anti-inflammatory properties, which may help with muscle soreness and recovery. It is thought to possibly be able to help with exercise intensity.

Exercise may be slightly impaired when progesterone and estrogen are both at their lowest point in the menstrual cycle. During the luteal phases, exercise capacity may be decreased. This means that cardio exercises like hiking may feel harder. Some females also experience decreased coordination and reaction times, and decreased ability to regulate body temperature. Exercising in the heat may feel more difficult.

You should be aware of the menstrual cycle and its possible effects on performance, but this doesn't mean you need to alter your plans just because you are in a certain phase of your cycle. Usually, just being aware of how your body feels and adjusting accordingly is all that needs to happen.

It's a good idea to track your cycle. This helps you be aware of when you will get your period, and also any symptoms associated with it. This can also give you information to assess whether you miss a period (amenorrhea) or your cycle length becomes too long (more than 35 days is called oligomenorrhea). This is a red flag that needs to be investigated. It could be a sign of pregnancy, polycystic ovarian syndrome, relative energy deficiency in sport (REDs), or something else. Some common period tracking apps are Fitr Woman, Flo, Apple Health, and Clue. There are many options available. For more on REDs see Chapter 6.

Some females may need to supplement with calcium and iron. Calcium may be needed to maintain bone health. Iron may be needed if menstrual blood losses are heavy or if you are anemic or deficient, which is common in female athletes. Check with your doctor to see if this is appropriate for you.

PREGNANT ATHLETES

Each pregnancy is different and carries with it the potential for various risks and complications. It is vital to get a physician to monitor your pregnancy to make sure both you and the baby are healthy. If you are cleared for exercise, the type of exercise, volume, and intensity will likely need to change over the course of your pregnancy. For example, skiing in early pregnancy may be totally fine, but not in the last semester when falling may put the baby's health at risk and your center of gravity is off.

Most females need additional folate (easily gotten from most prenatal vitamins), additional calories (between 300 and 450 per day), and more sleep. Eating foods rich in calcium, vitamin D, iron, and folate will help you and your baby's health. Folate is especially important in the period immediately after conception. Include adequate fluid and avoid foods that may cause foodborne illness, such as raw/undercooked meat and eggs, and soft cheeses.

MENOPAUSAL ATHLETES

Perimenopause and menopause can cause changes in body composition, with less lean mass and more fat mass distribution around the midsection. There can also be increased insulin resistance and decreased bone mineral density. To combat these changes, continue to exercise regularly, include strength training in your routine, and increase protein intake as needed. Aiming for about 40 grams per meal is a good goal. Also, try to be mindful of your energy intake versus energy expenditure, and don't eat more than your body needs. This is all easier said than done! It may be frustrating to see body composition changes when it feels like you haven't changed your exercise routine or diet. Checking with your doctor to see if hormone replacement therapy is right for you can be helpful in managing menopause symptoms.

PARA/ADAPTIVE ATHLETES

There are many types of para-athletes, and if you are reading this section, you likely are a para-athlete and know more than anyone else what your nutrition needs are. Depending on the category, different nutrition strategies may be used.

In general, most adaptive athletes need more calories during an active workout than other athletes. This is because movements may be less efficient. Adaptive athletes usually take more snacks and high-calorie foods with them, such as nut butter, sandwiches, and trail mix.

WHEELCHAIR ATHLETES

It's helpful to consult with a sports nutrition professional to figure out your specific nutrition needs. You can also use the concept of *metabolic equivalents* to estimate how many calories your body may need. A metabolic equivalent, or MET, is the amount of energy (measured in calories) your body needs per minute while resting quietly.

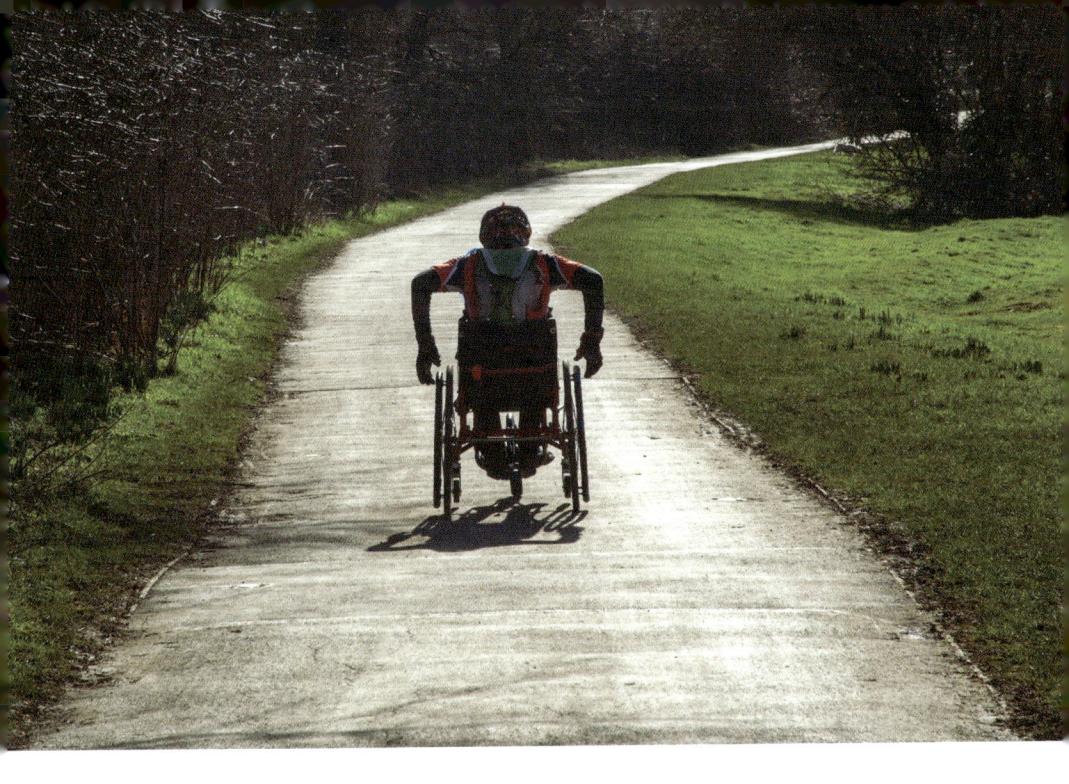

There are published tables that describe how many calories per minute certain wheelchair activities require. Called the Wheelchair Compendium of Physical Activities, it's a treasure trove of information that may be helpful to nail your nutrition needs.

Here's how it works: The Compendium lists various activities in METS. For example, fishing/casting is 1.1 METS, which is considered a "light" activity. If you wanted to estimate how many calories you burn while fishing for 1 hour, and you weighed 70 kilograms, you would calculate it with the following equation:

SOME METS FOR OTHER COMMON WHEELCHAIR SPORTS

11.8	Nordic sit skiing
1.8	Power wheelchair soccer
4.5	Handcycle racing
2.1	Resistance training
7.9	Wheeling—racing
2.6	Wheeling—outside
4.0	Wheeling—incline

Exercise calories = (MET level of activity × 3.5 × weight (kg) × minutes of activity) / 200 = calories burned per hour while doing that activity

So your total fishing calories = (1.1 METS × 3.5 × 70 kg × 60 minutes) / 200 = 81 calories per hour.

3 / SPECIAL NUTRITION SITUATIONS

This might be a helpful way to dial in on your fueling, but also be sure to have the basics down—eating regularly, hydrating regularly, and paying attention to body signals like hunger and fullness.

SPINAL INJURIES

Movement and sensory function may be altered or disrupted. Some people experience decreased cardiovascular capacity, decreased muscle mass, decreased sweat or body temperature regulation, decreased gastric emptying, and decreased resting metabolic rate.

Practical strategies could include being aware of sweat rate and replacing fluid losses as needed, keeping cool when possible by using light clothing, staying in the shade, or using cooling towels. In cold temperatures, using layered clothing and drinking hot liquids can help as well.

Try having snacks and fueling options on hand at all times. Snacks that are lower in fiber—or liquid calories—would be a good strategy for anyone struggling with slow gastric emptying. If you have compromised bowel or bladder control, working with a dietitian or keeping a food diary may be helpful to determine your own fluid needs, and which foods you tolerate that help facilitate normal bowel movements and keep to a bowel schedule.

BRAIN INJURIES AND CEREBRAL PALSY

People may struggle with difficulty with balance, posture, range of motion, and muscle coordination. They also may experience decreased sensation, cognition, and ability to communicate.

Nutrition strategies include matching energy intake with energy expenditure. This may take a bit of trial and error or working with a dietitian to make sure you are fueling yourself properly. If you are at risk for lower bone density (such as being in a wheelchair) pay attention to calcium and vitamin D intake and make sure you are getting correct amounts.

Some people may also experience swallowing difficulties and need special texture diets. Working closely with a speech therapist and dietitian will be useful to get ideas and make sure you are meeting your nutrient needs.

AMPUTEES

Like all other athletes, it's important to match energy intake to energy expenditure. This can be tricky as it ranges greatly from person to person. Working with a dietitian can help you nail this down. If you have a prosthesis, pressure wounds are a risk. You can mitigate this risk with good hygiene at the site, adequate overall calories, and adequate fluids. This helps support healthy skin structure.

Body composition techniques like a DEXA machine or BIA machine will not be accurate for an amputee. Instead, have a trained clinician take skinfold measurements if you need to monitor or manipulate body composition.

* * *

Each person has unique nutrition needs, and there is no exception for adaptive athletes. Find a dietitian that can help you optimize your nutrition for your particular situation. Use your own wisdom and experience to inform the process.

TRAVELING NUTRITION

If you're lucky, your outdoor adventures will take you to some places far from home. There are some nutrition tips you can apply to make your travels a success.

TRAVELING BY AIR

Most plane cabins are pressurized to the equivalent of around 6,000–8,000 feet elevation. This means you are exposed to high elevation even in the plane. If you live somewhere closer to sea level, this may put a stressor on your body.

Planes also usually have dry air, and more body fluid is lost through respiration in plane cabins than under normal circumstances. To manage these two factors, be sure to drink regularly on the plane ride. About 8 ounces every hour should be sufficient. This is especially important if you usually get headaches on flights, which may be caused by dehydration. You can consider adding electrolytes if it helps your body feel better, or if it helps you drink enough because of the flavoring. Avoid alcohol on the plane, as this will thwart hydration. Landing in a well-hydrated state may also be important if you are going to be in action as soon as you land. If you are expecting your body to hike or climb after landing, pre-hydrate and pre-fuel on the plane ride.

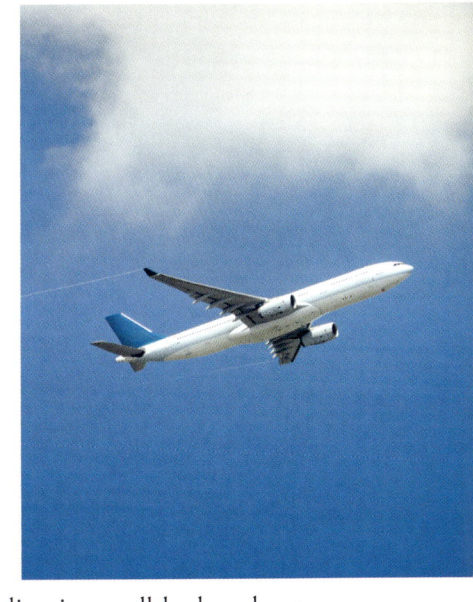

CROSSING TIME ZONES

This can wreak havoc on your sleep schedule. A few tips should keep the jet lag at bay:

- Try to match your sleep schedule to the new time zone as closely as possible.
- Minimize napping where possible to allow your body to adjust to the new bedtime.
- Consider using caffeine in the morning of your new time zone to train your body that it's time to be awake. Usual doses are anywhere from 40 milligrams to 200 milligrams.
- Consider using melatonin about an hour before bedtime in your new time zone to let your body know it's time to sleep. Usual doses are 1 milligram to 5 milligrams.
- Bring a sleep mask and earplugs. This helps block out light and sound to enable a good night's sleep.

TRAVEL SNACKS

Always bring snacks and water with you. Traveling is unpredictable. You never know if a flight will be delayed, your luggage will be lost, your taxi will never arrive, or your car will break down. Having an emergency stash of goodies on hand is a travel essential. Some ideas for your travel snacks:

- Trail mix and nuts
- Dried fruit and fruit leather
- Protein bars and powder mixes
- Water
- Shelf-stable juice, milk, or protein shakes
- Smoothie and applesauce pouches
- Pretzels and crackers
- Granola bars and energy bars
- Gummies and chocolate
- Dried snap peas and edamame
- Cup noodles
- Instant oatmeal
- Single-serve microwaveable mac and cheese or rice
- Nut butter pouches
- Jerky

Make sure you check the rules of entry if you are traveling to a different country. Some restrict foods brought from other countries.

AVOIDING FOOD POISONING

If you will be in an area with different sanitation standards than what you're used to, you may need to take some steps to avoid food poisoning. Drink only bottled water, avoid ice, and brush your teeth with bottled water. Avoid street vendors and restaurants as needed. If you become ill, you may need to seek medical treatment especially if you are experiencing vomiting and diarrhea, as you are at high risk for dehydration. Use caution when enjoying new foods.

NUTRITION FOR INJURY AND SURGERY

An injury is never in anyone's plans. It can really ruin a good season of adventuring! You may be able to prevent some injuries with the correct nutrition. If the injury has already occurred, you can help support the healing process.

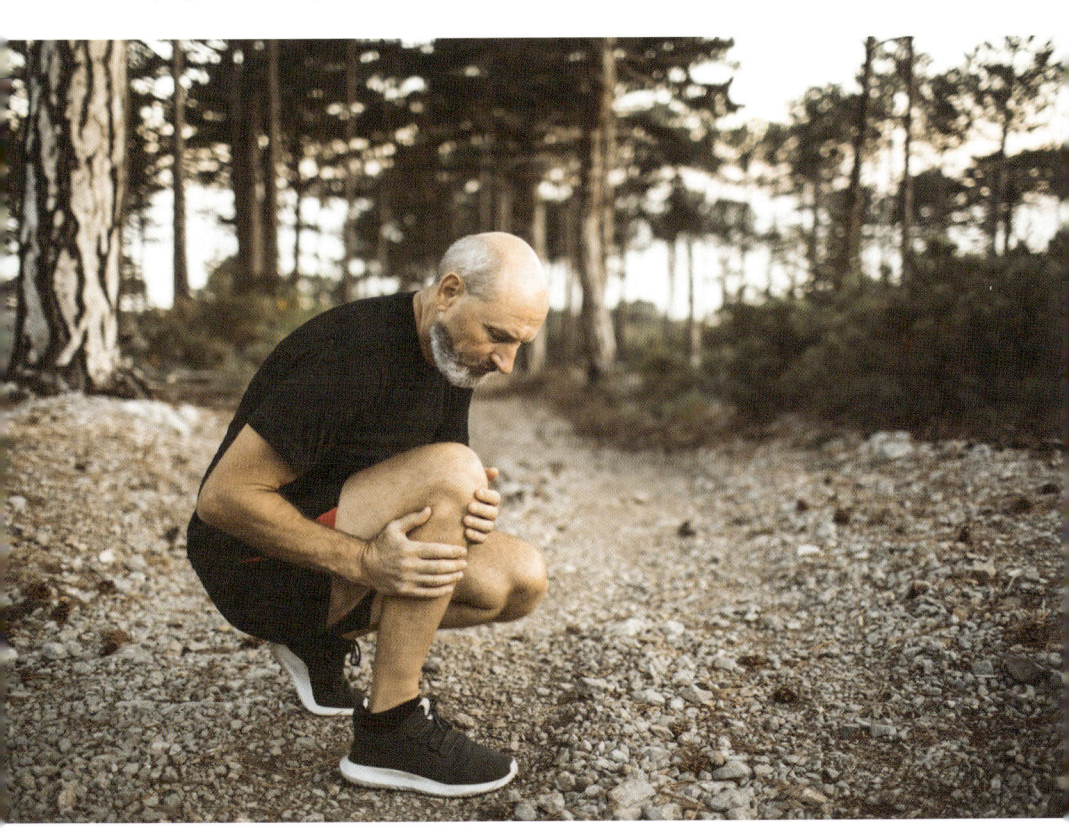

HOW NUTRITION CAN PREVENT INJURIES

Chronic injuries

These are injuries that take months to heal. Chronic injuries are complex and may be caused by a variety of factors, some of which are out of your control. There is a greater injury risk for those who chronically under-eat. If you have been on multiple diets, have a history of disordered eating, or inadvertently under-eat because you are so active, you may be at greater risk for injury.

Adequate overall calories, protein, carbohydrate, and many micronutrients support healthy tissues in your body. Think of all the different types of tissues—bone, intestines, organs, skin, ligaments, tendons, muscle—they all are active, living tissue that uses energy to maintain proper functioning and structure. If you under-eat, you are missing out on precious energy those tissues need. This coupled with heavy workouts or intense outdoor sports can put a big strain on these tissues. Tendons and ligaments may become weaker. Muscle mass declines. Bone density is compromised. Injury may result.

Acute Injuries

These are injuries that occur from a distinct event, such as falling and breaking a leg while hiking, or falling while skiing and breaking an arm. These injuries don't seem preventable—and in some cases, they aren't—but they *could* be in some instances.

Hear me out. Imagine you are climbing a multi-pitch route. You haven't been hydrating properly or eating regularly. You feel signs of low blood sugar—the shaky hands, the foggy mind, the irritability. You are tying a knot, or placing some trad gear, and you slip, fall, and break a bone. Oops—bummer, but preventable? What if you had eaten enough? Your mind would be clear. Your hands would be sure. Your mental game would be engaged.

In fact, dehydration and/or low blood sugar can manifest itself by:

- Decreased coordination
- Decreased concentration
- Missed shots
- Foggy mind
- Irritability

Acute injuries can sometimes be prevented by fueling and hydrating properly. Try to notice when your body feels fatigued, less coordinated, or less engaged in your activity. It may be time to take a break to eat and drink.

NUTRITION FOR INJURY AND SURGERY RECOVERY

Eat enough calories

It's tempting to decrease calorie intake when you're injured, especially if you are decommissioned for a bit and not doing your normal activities. However, your body needs extra calories to complete the healing process. It is increasing inflammation (in this case, that's a good thing that is part of healing). It is building up new tissue that was destroyed. It needs enough energy to do its thing. How many calories you need is very specific to your situation. Ask a dietitian for personalized help.

Eat Enough Protein

Protein is a key nutrient used to repair damaged tissues. Most people will need between 1.6 and 2.5 grams/kilogram/day. Aim for at least 20–40 grams per meal. Again, ask your dietitian for help to determine your specific needs. For more information on food sources of protein, see Chapter 1.

Collagen is a certain type of protein that may be particularly helpful for tendon and ligament injuries, as well as bone injuries. While research seems mixed as to how helpful it is, if you have the budget to buy collagen, it may be worth supplementing until you are healed. Aim for 15–20 grams per day. If you have physical therapy as part of your recovery process, taking collagen about 30–60 minutes before your physical therapy session may help aid recovery, especially if you are trying to heal from ligament and tendon injuries. See Chapter 4 for more supplement information.

Eat Enough Fruits and Vegetables

They contain many nutrients involved with healing, including vitamin A, vitamin C, and zinc. Bonus: They have fiber, which can help with regular bowel movements if you are constipated due to pain medications or lack of activity. Aim for at least one to two servings with each meal. You do not need to supplement with specific vitamins. This will not speed up the healing process. Rather, support your whole body with a variety of colorful produce.

Calcium and Vitamin D

These may need to be supplemented if you have a bone injury. These two nutrients are involved with bone mineral formation. Check with your doctor to see if this is appropriate for you.

Fish Oil

This may be appropriate for head injuries and concussions. Some evidence has shown it to be helpful in aiding recovery. Three to four grams per day is a typical dose. Check with your doctor to see if this is a good idea, as it is contraindicated in some conditions and those taking blood thinners.

Creatine Monohydrate

This has a lot of research behind it for strength training, but new research is pointing toward creatine as a helpful supplement for brain injury and to help prevent muscle atrophy when your muscles are immobilized or injured. The usual dose is 10 grams per day for 2 weeks (the "loading" phase), then 3 to 5 grams per day thereafter (the "maintenance" phase).

Avoid Alcohol

This is always a good idea, since alcohol is a toxin. Alcohol can impair wound healing, interfere with eating other nutrients, and interact with medications.

THE WRAP-UP

Wherever your outdoor adventures take you, you may find yourself needing specialized nutrition strategies for high altitude, heat, cold, travel, injury, and more. Tailor your needs to your specific situation to support your health and enhance performance.

REFERENCES

Conger, S. A., S. D. Herrmann, E. A. Willis, T. E. Nightingale, J. R. Sherman, and B. E. Ainsworth. "2024 Wheelchair Compendium of Physical Activities: An Update of Activity Codes and Energy Expenditure Values." *Journal of Sport and Health Science* 13, no. 1 (January 2024), 18–23. doi: 10.1016/j.jshs.2023.11.003. PMID: 38242594; PMCID: PMC10818147.

Karpinski, C., and C. Rosenbloom. *Sports Nutrition: A Handbook for Professionals*. Chicago: Academy of Nutrition and Dietetics, 2017.

Kechijian, D. "Optimizing Nutrition for Performance at Altitude: A Literature Review." *Journal of Special Operations Medicine* 11, no. 1 (Winter 2011), 12–17. doi: 10.55460/LXQK-O2RD. PMID: 21455904.

Khodaee, M., H. L. Grothe, J. H. Seyfert, and K. VanBaak. "Athletes at High Altitude." *Sports Health* 8, no. 2 (March-April 2016), 126–32. doi: 10.1177/1941738116630948. PMID: 26863894; PMCID: PMC4789936.

Luks, A. M., P. S. Auerbach, L. Freer, C. K. Grissom, L. E. Keyes, S. E. McIntosh, G. W. Rodway, R. B. Schoene, K. Zafren, and P. H. Hackett. "Wilderness Medical Society Clinical Practice Guidelines for the Prevention and Treatment of Acute Altitude Illness: 2019 Update." *Wilderness and Environmental Medicine* 30, no. 4 suppl. (December 2019), S3–S18. doi: 10.1016/j.wem.2019.04.006. Epub 2019 Jun 24. PMID: 31248818.

Mangieri, H. *Fueling Young Athletes*. Champaign, IL: Human Kinetics, 2017.

McNulty, K. L., K. J. Elliott-Sale, E. Dolan, P. A. Swinton, P. Ansdell, S. Goodall, K. Thomas, and K. M. Hicks. "The Effects of Menstrual Cycle Phase on Exercise Performance in Eumenorrheic Women: A Systematic Review and Meta-Analysis." *Sports Medicine* 50, no. 10 (October 2020), 1813–27. doi: 10.1007/s40279-020-01319-3. PMID: 32661839; PMCID: PMC7497427.

Ross, M., and D. T. Martin. "Altitude, Cold and Heat," in L. Burke and V. Deakin (eds.), *Clinical Sports Nutrition*, 5th ed. Sydney, Australia: McGraw Hill, 2015, 767–91.

Saunders, P. U., L. A. Garvican-Lewis, R. F. Chapman, and J. D. Périard. "Special Environments: Altitude and Heat." *International Journal of Sport Nutrition and Exercise Metabolism* 29 (2019), 210–19.

Sims, S. T., C. M. Kerksick, A. E. Smith-Ryan, X. A. K. Janse de Jonge, K. R. Hirsch, S. M. Arent, S. J. Hewlings, S. M. Kleiner, E. Bustillo, J. L. Tartar, V. G. Starratt, R. B. Kreider, C. Greenwalt, L. I. Rentería, M. J. Ormsbee, T. A. VanDusseldorp, B. I. Campbell, D.S. Kalman, and J. Antonio. "International Society of Sports Nutrition Position Stand: Nutritional Concerns of the Female Athlete." *Journal of the International Society of Sports Nutrition* 20, no. 1 (December 2023). doi: 10.1080/15502783.2023.2204066. PMID: 37221858; PMCID: PMC10210857.

Stellingwerff, T., P. Peeling, L. A. Garvican-Lewis, R. Hall, A. E. Koivisto, I. A. Heikura, and L. M. Burke. "Nutrition and Altitude: Strategies to Enhance Adaptation, Improve Performance and Maintain Health: A Narrative Review." *Sports Medicine* 49, suppl. 2 (December 2019), 169–84. doi: 10.1007/s40279-019-01159-w. PMID: 31691928; PMCID: PMC6901429.

Viscor, G., J. Corominas, and A. Carceller, "Nutrition and Hydration for High-Altitude Alpinism: A Narrative Review." *International Journal of Environmental Research and Public Health* 20 (2023), 3186. doi: 10.3390/ijerph20043186.

Yanagisawa, K., O. Ito, S. Nagi, and O. Shohei. "Electrolyte-Carbohydrate Beverage Prevents Water Loss in the Early Stage of High Altitude Training." *Journal of Medical Investigation* 59 (2011), 102–10.

4
SUPPLEMENTS

INTRODUCTION

The supplement industry is massive and unregulated. In 2021, it was estimated to be worth $152 billion. By 2028, it is estimated to be worth almost twice that at $300 billion. There are thousands upon thousands of products out there. Most are useless, some may be harmful, and only a few have research to support their efficacy and safety for enhancing sports performance.

The term *supplement* is a loose one. It usually means adding to, or "supplementing" your diet with another substance. A wordy-but-useful definition is "products containing concentrated sources of nutrients or other substances such as vitamins, minerals, botanicals, algae, fungi, bacteria, synthetic products, products of animal origin, amino acids, metabolites, etc., that are intended to supplement one's diet and have a nutritional or physiological effect, either alone or in combination with other substances."

Some people think of pills when they imagine supplements, but it could also mean a protein powder or a single-serve carbohydrate gel. For the purposes of this chapter, I will be talking about non-food supplements, such as creatine and beta-alanine, and discuss types of protein powders since these are so commonly used.

The list of evidence-based supplements that may help with sports performance is very short. We'll discuss each one in this chapter. As with all supplements, check with your doctor to make sure it is right for you before adding it to your routine.

Where do supplements fit into our goals from Chapter 1?

- Eat enough to support basic body processes.
- Eat enough to support training and movement (before, during, and after activity).
- Eat a healthful diet made of mostly whole grains, fruits/vegetables, nuts/seeds, dairy products, and lean protein.

- Refuel and rehydrate after workouts to promote recovery.
- Maintain a good relationship with food, body, and sport.

Supplements are just that—a *supplement* to a well-planned diet! They can support or enhance performance and health, but only if the foundation of an adequate diet is already in place.

HOW TO SELECT A SAFE SUPPLEMENT

Supplements are unregulated, which means they can contain banned substances (such as ephedra, steroids, or prohormones) and contaminants (such as lead and melamine), and you don't know if what is in the bottle is disclosed on the label. You also can't trust the label to give you the correct amounts or ingredients. In a scientific review article on supplements, it was found that 28 percent of all supplements that were tested in their sample size of 3,132 were contaminated with substances that could lead to a positive doping blood test.

To keep yourself safe, be sure to only use third-party tested supplements. Look for the USP logo, the NSF Certified for Sport seal, or the Informed Sport or Informed Choice logo.

Third-party tested supplements mean they have been batch-tested to detect contaminants and banned substances. Third-party testing is reassurance that their product would not trigger a positive doping test for elite athletes. I recommend using third-party tested supplements no matter who you are, because even if you are not subject to doping tests, you don't want to be ingesting contaminants or banned substances.

While third-party testing is useful, it does not mean the supplement is worthwhile or evidence based. A supplement may be "clean" but ineffective. Also of note: Just because something is "natural" doesn't mean it is safe. Be sure you understand the supplement you are taking—does it interact with any other supplements or medications you are taking? Is it contraindicated for certain health conditions? Use caution.

Remember our pyramid from Chapter 2?

Supplements are at the top of the pyramid because they are the least important. They may give you an edge, but if nutrition is not in place, supplements cannot fix the problem of a poorly nourished body.

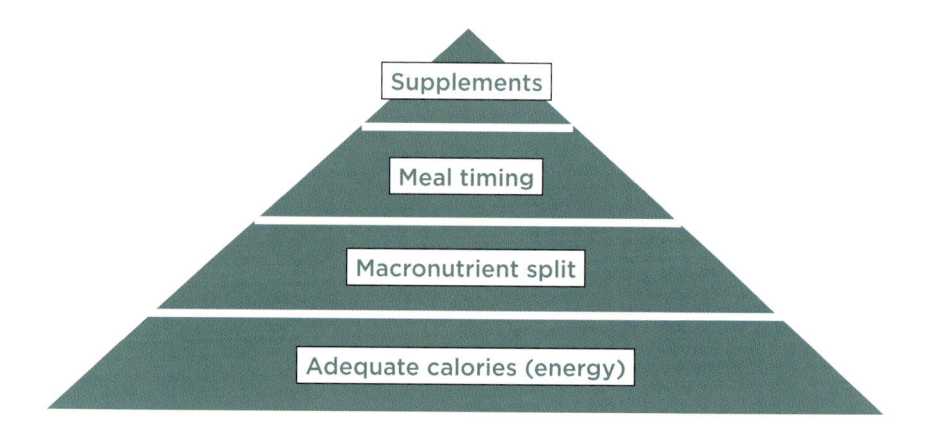

Pyramid (bottom to top): Adequate calories (energy); Macronutrient split; Meal timing; Supplements

Before taking a supplement, ask yourself these questions:

- Is it safe?
- Is it third-party tested?
- Is it legal?
- Do I understand what it is supposed to do for me?
- Is it effective?
- Do I understand the proper dosing and timing?
- Did I get my information from a reliable source, such as a sports dietitian (not a coach or friend)?
- Do I have everything else in place, such as nutrition, hydration, rest days, and sleep?
- Do I have the budget for it?

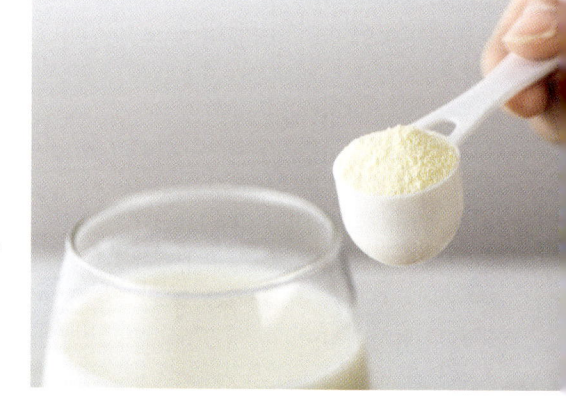

Use caution and speak with your doctor and dietitian before adding supplements. This can keep you safe and save a lot of money.

Now read on for more information about supplements that may be worth considering.

CREATINE

Creatine is one of the most widely researched and safe supplements out there. Your body actually makes creatine, but it is helpful to supplement in some situations. Creatine is found in meat, but not in large enough amounts to make a notable difference in performance.

WHAT IT DOES

Creatine is involved with the adenosine triphosphate-phosphocreatine system (ATP-PC system). (See Chapter 1 for a refresher on this energy system.) It can help increase the time to fatigue when doing short, intense movements like lifting weights. It is best for short-duration movements and maximum-intensity movements. This could feel like you can go a little longer or harder on movements such as sprints, climbing dynos, or ski tricks.

More recent research also shows promising implications for brain health. Creatine may be used after a head injury or concussion, and some other research shows it helps with cognition in older adults. It also has anti-inflammatory properties.

Taking creatine consistently may help you gain more lean muscle mass. This is because it enables a more effective workout. If you have a structured lifting program, combined with creatine, this may help build more muscle mass than lifting alone.

If you don't lift weights, you may still benefit from creatine, depending on your sport. Any sport that involves intense movements or short bursts of effort can benefit from creatine. There is evidence that even endurance athletes may benefit from creatine supplementation.

HOW TO TAKE IT

Since creatine is found in meat products, vegans and vegetarians may see a larger benefit from creatine supplementation than omnivores. A typical omnivore diet contains about 1–2 grams per day.

The recommended dosage for supplementation is 3 to 5 grams per day. You can start with a "loading protocol" of 20 grams per day for 5 to 7 days, then switch to a maintenance dose of 3 to 5 grams daily. Or you can skip the loading protocol and go straight to the maintenance dose. It will just take slightly longer for the muscles to become fully saturated with creatine.

It is tasteless and dissolves easily in liquid. Most people take it by mixing creatine powder into their coffee, water, sports drink, or protein shake. Take it daily. You do not need to overthink the timing. If you take it consistently every day, it will be effective.

Creatine monohydrate is the most studied form of creatine. It is also the cheapest. Some supplement companies will try to market other forms as being superior or helping avoid water weight gain, but these are more expensive and often less effective.

IMPORTANT NOTES

Since creatine is stored in the muscle with water molecules, some people notice weight gain when taking it. This is just water weight and will shed off with exercise. You may gain between 1 and 5 pounds.

Some people experience gastrointestinal symptoms with creatine. If this is the case with you, try dividing it up into smaller doses and take multiple times per day.

Use caution if you have existing kidney disease. It may not be appropriate for you. As with all supplements, ask your doctor before taking creatine.

BETA-ALANINE

Beta-alanine is an amino acid. Like creatine, it is produced in your body and found in the diet, but supplementation may help with sports performance.

WHAT IT DOES

Beta-alanine acts as a buffer in the skeletal muscle. Think back to a time when you had a burning sensation in your muscles. This may have happened to your calves while walking up a steep trail, or to your thighs while skiing down a mountain. The burning can be alleviated or lessened with beta-alanine. Some people find it useful, especially if the burning sensation is what limits their activity. For example, burning in the forearms while climbing may cause you to pause or stop climbing for a bit. Imagine if you didn't have that acute burning sensation!

This supplement can increase the time to fatigue and reduce the burning in your muscles. This may translate into better sports performance if it enables you to go longer or harder. It's most useful for exercises lasting around 30 seconds to 10 minutes.

HOW TO TAKE IT

The normal dose of beta-alanine is 4 to 6 grams daily, divided into two doses.

Taking it with meals is helpful. Use it daily for best results. You may consider taking it about 15–30 minutes before a workout, but as long as you take it daily at about the same time, you should be able to notice benefits. Most research has studied its effects between 4 and 10 weeks. It is unknown if long-term beta-alanine supplementation is useful or safe.

Like creatine, it is sold in a powder form and mixed with liquid. Beta-alanine is a common ingredient in commercial pre-workout supplement blends.

IMPORTANT NOTES

It may be beneficial to take alongside sodium bicarbonate. See the next section for more information on this supplement.

Beta-alanine may cause a tingling sensation, called paraesthesia. It is harmless, but some people find it annoying. This is why it is split into two doses each day. A full dose of 4 to 6 grams taken at one time may not be as effective.

A well-trained athlete in peak physical condition may not benefit from beta-alanine as much as an untrained athlete. If you try it, check with your doctor first and experiment to see if you notice any usefulness.

SODIUM BICARBONATE

You may be surprised to hear that sodium bicarbonate is good ol' baking soda. The cheapest of all the supplements, you can get a dose of sodium bicarbonate for pennies. It's probably in your kitchen right now!

WHAT IT DOES

Sodium bicarbonate may help with that burning sensation in your muscles that occurs when you are working hard. It acts as a buffer, similar to beta-alanine. It may increase power and time to exhaustion, and reduce fatigue. It is most useful for short bouts of high-intensity effort. It can also help with endurance sports such as mountain biking, trail running, or competitive rowing where effort is intense for a long duration. It is most useful for events lasting between 30 seconds and 12 minutes.

HOW TO TAKE IT

If you want the cheap version, you mix baking soda with 16 ounces of water and sip it slowly over the course of 60–90 minutes before your workout. The recommended dose is 0.3 gram/kilogram of body weight.

This would look like:

3.5 teaspoons for a 100-pound person
4 teaspoons for a 120-pound person
5 teaspoons for a 150-pound person
6 teaspoons for a 180-pound person
6.75 teaspoons for a 200-pound person

There is also a loading protocol where you can take it over the course of 5 days, although research is mixed as to how effective this is.

There are also commercial capsules available. This bypasses the step of drinking bitter water before your workout, but may require you to take several capsules with water, depending on the brand you choose. Another form available is in a gel, which is quite expensive and not well studied to determine its effectiveness.

IMPORTANT NOTES

As with all supplements, weighing the risk versus the benefit is important. Sodium bicarbonate is known to cause gastrointestinal upset. Many people experience bloating, nausea, stomach pain, and even diarrhea. If you think sodium bicarbonate may be useful for you, test it in controlled conditions first. Try it during a home workout or at the gym—somewhere near a bathroom and on a day when you can stop working out easily if something goes wrong. Do not try this for the first time in the backcountry. That's good advice for any new supplement!

Taking it with a meal may help reduce these side effects. Trying it in smaller doses three to four times per day, and taking it in capsule form may also help.

CAFFEINE

This is likely the most widely used supplement, as it is found in many common food items. Many people worldwide ingest caffeine regularly in coffee, tea, sodas, chocolate, energy drinks, and other drinks like yerba mate and guarana. It's also found in engineered sports products such as gummies, gels, gum, and beverages.

WHAT IT DOES

You've probably known firsthand what it does in your body! Sports performance research shows that this stimulant can improve cognition, reaction time, coordination, neuromuscular function, and alertness, and reduce the perception of fatigue and pain during exercise.

It may help with jumping, sprinting, endurance activities, strength movements, throwing movements, and more. It may also help give an extra boost at high altitudes or extreme heat.

Caffeine can be beneficial for all sorts of outdoor activities. From long thru-hikes to short ski runs and everything in between, caffeine can help you feel better.

HOW TO TAKE IT

Caffeine comes in many forms. Use caution that you don't take too much in 1 day inadvertently. Since it is so common, it can be easy to get too much. Be aware of all the sources you may be ingesting in a day, including energy drinks, coffee, soda, sports gummies, and more.

The dose most research recommends for sports performance enhancement is 3–6 milligrams per kilogram of body weight, taken about 60 minutes before exercise. This is around 200 milligrams for many people. You may feel a nice effect with even less than this. Take it with a carbohydrate for an even better pre-workout boost.

IMPORTANT NOTES

Caffeine does cause stomach upset in some people. If you notice a lot of bloating or diarrhea, you may not want to take this, especially if you're in the backcountry. While it is a diuretic, it doesn't dehydrate you. It does, however, stimulate the bladder in some people, which creates the urge to urinate. If your preferred method of caffeine ingestion is a liquid, you may need to urinate more simply because you are drinking more fluid. Research suggests that even up to 4 cups of coffee can still contribute to your overall fluid needs for the day without undue diuretic effects.

Use caution with too much caffeine. If you have a heart condition, ask your doctor first about the right amount (if any) for you. It can cause withdrawal symptoms such as headaches and irritability. It can also cause symptoms like a jittery feeling, anxiety, high blood pressure, and a fast heartbeat.

Be careful when taking it too close to bedtime, as it can interfere with the onset of sleep as well as the quality of sleep. Most recommendations suggest using caffeine no later than 1–3 p.m. for best sleep outcomes.

Supplement	Uses	Dose	Notes
Creatine	Short, intense efforts	3–5 g daily	May cause water weight gain. Avoid if you have kidney disease.
Beta-alanine	Short, intense efforts	4–6 g daily divided into two doses	May cause tingling sensation
Sodium bicarbonate	Short, intense efforts	0.3 g/kg of body weight	May cause gastrointestinal issues
Caffeine	Most activities can benefit from caffeine use.	200 mg or 0.3 g/kg body weight 60 minutes before exercise	May cause gastrointestinal issues, headaches, anxiety, and interfere with sleep
Beet juice	Endurance activities	2.5 ounces taken 90 minutes before the workout	Avoid if you have kidney stones
Omega-3 fatty acids	Muscle soreness, performance enhancement, concussion recovery	1,000–4,000 mg daily	Check with your doctor to make sure it is safe for you
Collagen	Joint and soft tissue health	10–20 g daily	Mixed research as to effectiveness

BEET JUICE

Beet juice contains a substance called nitrates. Nitrates sound scary. Isn't that the thing in cured meats that may cause cancer in large doses? Um, yes, however, nitrates are plentiful in fruits and vegetables. When they are sourced from these foods, they may have a positive health outcome. Fruits and vegetables may reduce cancer risk. Nitrates in a sports supplement context are found in beet juice products.

WHAT IT DOES

But what does all this have to do with sports performance? Nitrates in food or a beet juice shot can increase levels of nitric oxide in the blood. This, in turn, can increase blood flow, strengthen muscle contractions, and improve gas exchange within the blood (oxygen and carbon dioxide). Some studies show athletes have greater cardiorespiratory efficiency and endurance, they can go longer until fatigue, and they have improved VO_2 max. Studies are mixed, and the effectiveness of nitrate supplementation depends on the fitness of the individual and the dose of nitrates the beet juice actually contains.

HOW TO TAKE IT

You can simply add more high-nitrate vegetables to your diet, including leafy green veggies, celery, and beets. You can also use commercially prepared supplements such as beet root shots or beet powder mixed with water.

You can try 2.5 ounces of beet juice concentrate about 90 minutes before your workout. You need to take it for about 5 days in a row in order to see benefits. Some studies show that taking it for 12 days in a row before the event is beneficial.

IMPORTANT NOTES

Nitrites can begin to be broken down while exposed to saliva in the mouth. The bacteria in your mouth helps convert them from nitrites to nitrates (a normal body process). However, if you have killed all the bacteria in your mouth with mouthwash, this process will not occur, thereby rendering your special beet root shot mostly useless.

Based on current research, it also seems that the performance-enhancing effects of beet juice may be slim to none in a very well-trained individual. Elite athletes at the top of their game see less benefit than untrained people. This is likely because the elite athlete already has a lot of useful body adaptations to maximize performance and efficiency that an untrained person doesn't have yet. Beet juice can give this untrained person more of an edge.

Avoid beet juice if you have a history of kidney stones. Nitrate can bind with calcium in the body and form a kidney stone.

Beet juice may help with performance at high altitudes. Studies are mixed, but it could be useful to take, or at least include green leafy vegetables in your high-altitude adventure menu where possible.

FISH OIL/OMEGA-3S

Omega-3 fatty acids, found in fish oil, have gained a lot of attention over the years for their implications in heart health and their anti-inflammatory properties. You can get these fatty acids from food sources like fatty fish, nuts and seeds, flaxseed, soybean, and canola oils (although plant sources are not used in your body as effectively). Omega-3s can also be found in eggs if the chickens are given a special feed.

WHAT IT DOES

Fish oil may reduce muscle soreness, reduce tissue damage from exercise, increase endurance capacity, reduce illness risk, and help with concussion recovery. It may also help with mood and cognition. Study findings are mixed.

HOW TO TAKE IT

Include fatty fish in your diet (salmon, mackerel, cod, herring, sardines, and anchovies) two to three times per week. Alternatively, you can take a fish oil supplement. Most studies have suggested doses of 1,000–4,000 milligrams daily. Be sure your supplement is third-party tested. Impurities abound in fish oil supplements, particularly heavy metals.

IMPORTANT NOTES

Vegans and vegetarians can take algal oil instead of fish oil. If you are interested in taking a fish oil supplement, first ask your doctor. Your diet may be adequate already. Also, fish oil should not be taken with blood thinners.

COLLAGEN

Collagen has seen some really convincing marketing in the past few years. The claims are convincing, but the research is mixed.

Collagen is a type of protein found in tendons, ligaments, and bone. It is usually sold in powder or capsule form. The capsules are usually marketed toward hair, skin, and nail health in doses lower than what you would need for soft tissue health like tendon or ligament repair and joint health or recovery from injury.

WHAT IT DOES

Collagen may help thicken cartilage and tendons/ligaments. It may also help reduce joint pain. Some studies show people report less knee pain when they use collagen consistently. It may also help with skin and bone health, especially after an injury or surgery. There are many promising claims, but the actual research is more nuanced and mixed.

HOW TO TAKE IT

For best outcomes, skip the low-dose capsule and use collagen powder. The therapeutic dose is between 10 and 15 grams per day based on current research. You can mix it with any drink, as it is tasteless and combines well with fluids. Many people put it in their coffee or smoothies.

If you are trying to support tendon and ligament health, taking it about 30 minutes before your workout can be helpful. This allows the collagen to get into the bloodstream and be taken up by the soft tissues where enhanced blood flow is occurring during the workout.

Some studies have paired collagen with vitamin C, because this is a vitamin involved with soft tissue structure. You can take 5–50 milligrams of vitamin C with your collagen, or simply mixing it into orange juice will also do the trick.

IMPORTANT NOTES

Since it is simply a protein and has minimal (if any) side effects or risks, I usually recommend taking collagen only if you have your diet dialed in, you have the budget for it, you are eating enough protein and calories, and you have a reason to take it (such as joint problems or a torn ligament). If adequate nutrition is not in place, collagen may not do much for you. Eating enough calories and protein is much more impactful to muscle and bone health than a collagen supplement.

Collagen is missing a few key amino acids for optimal muscle building and recovery, so do not view collagen as an optimal protein powder supplement (more about protein powders in the next section).

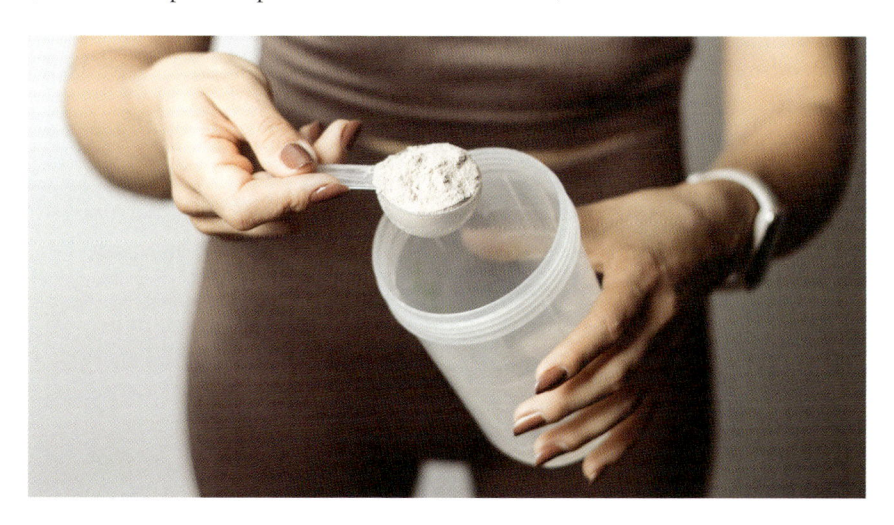

This is not a vegan or vegetarian product. There are supplements on the market calling themselves "vegan collagen," but it is usually just a selection of some vitamins and minerals. This is not a valid collagen substitute. Don't waste your money.

PROTEIN POWDERS

Protein powders are not necessary, but can be very convenient for the outdoor athlete. Backpackers find them useful to get nutrition on the trail in a lightweight packet. They can be used to help you reach your daily protein goals if it seems too hard to get it from food alone. Protein powders are also useful if you need to nourish your body but don't have time or access to a full meal.

A "complete protein" means that it contains all amino acids. A full complement of amino acids is useful for muscle rebuilding and repair, as well as numerous body processes.

You do not need branched-chain amino acids (BCAAs). These are hyped up and well marketed, but largely useless. If your diet is adequate in overall protein, don't waste your money on BCAAs.

HOW TO TAKE IT

Protein powders are easily mixed with water, milk, plant "milks," smoothies, oatmeal, yogurt, soup, and more. The options are endless, and they can really come in handy when you are backpacking or camping. There are also many shelf-stable ready-to-drink shakes on the market.

In general, aim for about 20–40 grams of protein per serving. Your individual protein needs will vary. You should be getting protein from your diet as well, so how often you use a protein supplement will depend on what other source of protein you are eating throughout the day.

IMPORTANT NOTES

As with all supplements, make sure your protein powder is third-party tested. Some protein powders have been contaminated with lead, mercury, hormones, steroids, and banned substances.

There are many types of protein on the market. Here is a guide to help you choose which one is right for you.

PICK A PROTEIN POWDER

Type of Powder	Definition	Qualities	Complete Protein?
Whey hydrolysate	"Pre-digested," broken down whey isolate particles for quick digestion	Easily digested, high-protein source with quality amino acids, contains lactose	Yes
Whey isolate	Pure form of whey protein. Filtered from cow's milk. Usually about 90% protein.	High-protein source with quality amino acids, low lactose	Yes
Whey concentrate	Less filtered than whey isolate—some carbohydrates still present from natural sugars (lactose) in the milk. Usually about 70–80% protein.	Good protein source. Contains lactose.	Yes
Casein	Another milk protein	Slowly digested. Best for right before bedtime. Contains lactose.	Yes
Pea	From ground peas with the fiber and starch removed	Slowly digested. Good vegan option.	No
Soy	From ground soybeans	Good vegan option	Yes
Hemp	From the hemp plant (not marijuana)	Use caution—may contain trace amounts of THC, which would cause a positive doping test. Higher in fiber, slowly digested.	Yes
Collagen protein	Made from bones, skin, and cartilage of animals	May help with soft tissue injuries	No
Plant protein blend (soy, pea, hemp, etc.)	From ground plant proteins	May have better amino acid profile due to a variety of plants used. Good vegan option. Not superior to whey.	Depends on the blend, but whey is still likely higher in leucine
Egg	Made from dehydrated chicken eggs	Easily absorbed and digested	Yes

THE WRAP-UP

Supplements can be a useful addition to the outdoor athlete's diet. Very few are well researched. Since they have very little regulation, use caution when adding a supplement to your diet. Look for third-party testing and check with your health care professional to make sure it is appropriate for you. Some supplements may interact with medications.

REFERENCES

Antonio, J., D. E. Newmire, J. R. Stout, B. Antonio, M. Gibbons, L. M. Lowery, J. Harper, D. Willoughby, C. Evans, D. Anderson, E. Goldstein, J. Rojas, M. Monsalves-Álvarez, S. C. Forbes, J. Gomez Lopez, T. Ziegenfuss, B. D. Moulding, D. Candow, M. Sagner, and S. M. Arent. "Common Questions and Misconceptions About Caffeine Supplementation: What Does the Scientific Evidence Really Show?" *Journal of the International Society of Sports Nutrition* 21, no. 1 (December 2024), 2323919. doi: 10.1080/15502783.2024.2323919. Epub 2024 Mar 11. PMID: 38466174; PMCID: PMC10930107.

Butts, J., B. Jacobs, and M. Silvis. "Creatine Use in Sports." *Sports Health* 10, no. 1 (January/February 2018), 31–34. doi: 10.1177/1941738117737248. Epub 2017 Oct 23. PMID: 29059531; PMCID: PMC5753968.

Djaoudene, O., A. Romano, Y. D. Bradai, F. Zebiri, A. Ouchene, Y. Yousfi, M. Amrane-Abider, Y. Sahraoui-Remini, and K. Madani. "A Global Overview of Dietary Supplements: Regulation, Market Trends, Usage during the COVID-19 Pandemic, and Health Effects." *Nutrients* 15, no. 15 (July 26, 2023), 3320. doi: 10.3390/nu15153320. PMID: 37571258; PMCID: PMC10421343.

Domínguez, R., E. Cuenca, J. L. Maté-Muñoz, P. García-Fernández, N. Serra-Paya, M. C. Estevan, P. V. Herreros, and M. V. Garnacho-Castaño. "Effects of Beetroot Juice Supplementation on Cardiorespiratory Endurance in Athletes. A Systematic Review." *Nutrients* 9, no. 1 (January 6, 2017), 43. doi: 10.3390/nu9010043. PMID: 28067808; PMCID: PMC5295087.

Forbes, S. C., D. G. Candow, J. H. F. Neto, M. D. Kennedy, J. L. Forbes, M. Machado, E. Bustillo, J. Gomez-Lopez, A. Zapata, and J. Antonio. "Creatine Supplementation and Endurance Performance: Surges and Sprints to Win the Race." *Journal of the International Society of Sports Nutrition* 20, no. 1 (December 2023), 2204071. doi: 10.1080/15502783.2023.2204071. PMID: 37096381; PMCID: PMC10132248.

Gammone, M. A., G. Riccioni, G. Parrinello, and N. D'Orazio. "Omega-3 Polyunsaturated Fatty Acids: Benefits and Endpoints in Sport." *Nutrients* 11, no. 1 (December 27, 2018), 46. doi: 10.3390/nu11010046. PMID: 30591639; PMCID: PMC6357022.

Grgic, J., Z. Pedisic, B. Saunders, G. G. Artioli, B. J. Schoenfeld, M. J. McKenna, D. J. Bishop, R. B. Kreider, J. R. Stout, D. S. Kalman, S. M. Arent, T. A. VanDusseldorp, H. L. Lopez, T. N. Ziegenfuss, L. M. Burke, J. Antonio, and B. I. Campbell. "International Society of Sports Nutrition Position Stand: Sodium Bicarbonate and Exercise Performance." *Journal of the International Society of Sports Nutrition* 18, no. 1 (September 9, 2021), 61. doi: 10.1186/s12970-021-00458-w. PMID: 34503527; PMCID: PMC8427947.

Guest, N. S., T. A. VanDusseldorp, M. T. Nelson, J. Grgic, B. J. Schoenfeld, N. D. M. Jenkins, S. M. Arent, J. Antonio, J. R. Stout, E. T. Trexler, A. E. Smith-Ryan, E. R. Goldstein, D. S. Kalman, and B. I. Campbell. "International Society of Sports Nutrition Position Stand: Caffeine and Exercise Performance." *Journal of the International Society of Sports Nutrition* 18 no. 1 (January 2, 2021), 1. doi: 10.1186/s12970-020-00383-4. PMID: 33388079; PMCID: PMC7777221.

Heileson, J. L., S. B. Machek, D. R. Harris, S. Tomek, L. C. de Souza, A. J. Kieffer, N. D. Barringer, A. Gallucci, J. S. Forsse, and L. K. Funderburk. "The Effect of Fish Oil Supplementation on Resistance Training–Induced Adaptations." *Journal of the International Society of Sports Nutrition* 20, no. 1 (December 2023), 2174704. doi: 10.1080/15502783.2023.2174704. PMID: 36822153; PMCID: PMC9970203.

Khatri, M., R. J. Naughton, T. Clifford, L. D. Harper, and L. Corr. "The Effects of Collagen Peptide Supplementation on Body Composition, Collagen Synthesis, and Recovery from Joint Injury and Exercise: A Systematic Review." *Amino Acids* 53, no. 10 (October 2021), 1493–1506. doi: 10.1007/s00726-021-03072-x. Epub 2021 Sep 7. PMID: 34491424; PMCID: PMC8521576.

Kozhuharov, V. R., K. Ivanov, and S. Ivanova. "Dietary Supplements as Source of Unintentional Doping." *Biomed Research International*, April 22, 2022, 8387271. doi: 10.1155/2022/8387271. PMID: 35496041; PMCID: PMC9054437.

Martínez-Sanz, J. M., I. Sospedra, C. M. Ortiz, E. Baladía, A. Gil-Izquierdo, and R. Ortiz-Moncada. "Intended or Unintended Doping? A Review of the

Presence of Doping Substances in Dietary Supplements Used in Sports." *Nutrients* 9, no. 10 (October 4, 2017), 1093. doi: 10.3390/nu9101093. PMID: 28976928; PMCID: PMC5691710.

Martinho, D. V., H. Nobari, A. Faria, A. Field, D. Duarte, and H. Sarmento. "Oral Branched-Chain Amino Acids Supplementation in Athletes: A Systematic Review." *Nutrients* 14, no. 19 (September 27, 2022), 4002. doi: 10.3390/nu14194002. PMID: 36235655; PMCID: PMC9571679.

Maughan, R. J., L. M. Burke, J. Dvorak, D. E. Larson-Meyer, P. Peeling, S. M. Phillips, E. S. Rawson, N. P. Walsh, I. Garthe, H. Geyer, R. Meeusen, L. J. C. van Loon, S. M. Shirreffs, L. L. Spriet, M. Stuart, A. Vernec, K. Currell, V. M. Ali, R. G. Budgett, A. Ljungqvist, M. Mountjoy, Y. P. Pitsiladis, T. Soligard, U. Erdener, and L. Engebretsen. "IOC Consensus Statement: Dietary Supplements and the High-Performance Athlete." *British Journal of Sports Medicine* 52, no. 7 (April 2018), 439–55. doi: 10.1136/bjsports-2018-099027. Epub 2018 Mar 14. PMID: 29540367; PMCID: PMC5867441.

Philpott, J. D., O. C. Witard, and S. D. R. Galloway. "Applications of Omega-3 Polyunsaturated Fatty Acid Supplementation for Sport Performance." *Research in Sports Medicine* 27, no. 2 (April–June 2019), 219–37. doi: 10.1080/15438627.2018.1550401. Epub 2018 Nov 28. PMID: 30484702.

Shannon, O. M., K. McGawley, L. Nybäck, L. Duckworth, M. J. Barlow, D. Woods, M. Siervo, and J. P. O'Hara. "'Beet-ing' the Mountain: A Review of the Physiological and Performance Effects of Dietary Nitrate Supplementation at Simulated and Terrestrial Altitude." *Sports Medicine* 47, no. 11 (November 2017), 2155–69. doi: 10.1007/s40279-017-0744-9. PMID: 28577258; PMCID: PMC5633647.

Thielecke, F., and A. Blannin. "Omega-3 Fatty Acids for Sport Performance—Are They Equally Beneficial for Athletes and Amateurs? A Narrative Review." *Nutrients* 12, no. 12 (November 30, 2020), 3712. doi: 10.3390/nu12123712. PMID: 33266318; PMCID: PMC7760705.

Trexler, E. T., A. E. Smith-Ryan, J. R. Stout, J. R. Hoffman, C. D. Wilborn, C. Sale, R. B. Kreider, R. Jäger, C. P. Earnest, L. Bannock, B. Campbell, D. Kalman, T. N. Ziegenfuss, and J. Antonio. "International Society of Sports Nutrition Position Stand: Beta-Alanine." *Journal of the International Society of Sports Nutrition* 12, no. 30 (July 15, 2015). doi: 10.1186/s12970-015-0090-y. PMID: 26175657; PMCID: PMC4501114.

5
FUELING YOUR ADVENTURE

Note: This book was designed for people to read only sections relevant to them. Some people may not read it cover-to-cover. Some information presented in previous sections and Chapter 3 will be presented here as well.

Welcome to the chapter all about individual sports! You still want to keep in mind our overarching goals:

- Eat enough to support basic body processes.
- Eat enough to support training and movement (before, during, and after activity).
- Eat a healthful diet made of mostly whole grains, fruits/vegetables, nuts/seeds, dairy products, and lean protein.
- Refuel and rehydrate after workouts to promote recovery.
- Maintain a good relationship with food, body, and sport.

These goals apply even to these sport-specific recommendations. But here, we'll get into the nitty-gritty of how to fuel and hydrate for most scenarios you may encounter in your outdoor fun.

Naomi had a great experience with learning how to fuel properly. My hope for you is that this section can provide solid information so you can have great outcomes too!

"I had one of my best climbing days ever because I was fueling consistently! I learned the importance of eating enough carbs throughout the climbing day as well as staying ahead of hunger. I started my day with a protein smoothie and a banana. Then I packed homemade granola bars, a bagel with honey, a banana, crackers, pretzels, apples, fruit snacks, as well as a protein shake for the car ride home. I ate throughout the day, before I was even hungry, and stayed hydrated, and had a great climbing day. I took my time resting between boulders and snacking, and then got my first V9 flash. I fueled properly the whole day with carbs and felt good. Because of my consistent fueling, I recovered quickly and was always ready for the next climbing day!"

Since each sport has unique fueling needs and challenges, your energy needs will vary widely depending on the sport, the environmental conditions, your own body characteristics (height, weight, age, gender, body composition), and the duration and intensity of the sport. For you to more accurately estimate your fueling needs, we can use the concept of *metabolic equivalents*, or METS.

A metabolic equivalent is the amount of energy (measured in calories) your body uses per minute while resting quietly. This was covered in other sections, but here is a refresher. You can use this equation to calculate your estimated energy expenditure during the duration of the activity.

$$\text{Exercise calories} = (\text{MET level of activity} \times 3.5 \times \text{weight (kg)} \times \text{minutes of activity}) / 200$$

Here is an example of a 70-kilogram snowboarder, with 3 hours of active snowboarding over the course of a day.

"Skiing, downhill, alpine or snowboarding, moderate effort, active time only" is 6.3 METS.

6.3 METS × 3.5 × 70 kg × 180 minutes/200 = 1,389 calories burned.

You will see METS listed in this chapter with each sport category. This will help you estimate your own energy expenditure for whatever sport you choose to do.

SNOW SPORTS

Welcome, winter athlete! We've already covered nutrition basics for cold weather in Chapter 3, but now we will take a deeper dive into the practical logistics. The principles and strategies in this section can be applied to most, if not all, snow sports.

HYDRATION

Winter athletes can lose up to 3 to 8 percent of their body weight during a workout due to water losses. Sweat and respiration make up a large part of this. Barriers to fluid intake include reduced thirst, limited fluid access (especially if it freezes), and purposefully skipping fluids to avoid urinating. This can decrease sports performance, and severe dehydration can be a medical emergency. High altitude puts an additional stressor on your body.

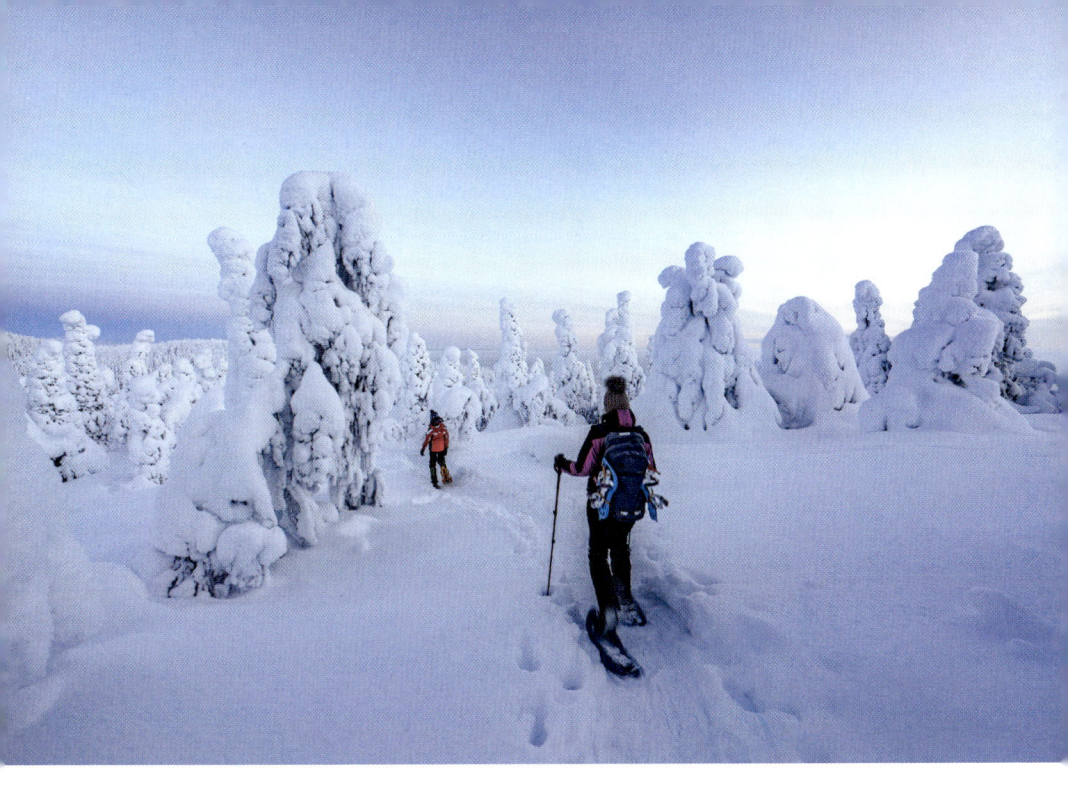

Amount	Types of Fluids	How to Carry	Tips
8–16 oz per hour	Water Sports drinks Soups Broth Hot chocolate Coffee Tea	Nalgene bottles Double-walled, insulated metal containers Bladder-hose system (if conditions are above freezing) Collapsible flasks (if conditions are above freezing) Carry close to body to prevent freezing if necessary	You may need more fluid depending on your sweat rate and the environmental conditions. If you lost more than 2–3% of your body weight, rehydrate with 16–24 oz sports drink after your workout. Female athletes can consider using a urinal device or pants with a full zipper fly (front to back) to allow for easy urination without prolonged cold exposure.

5 / FUELING YOUR ADVENTURE   **101**

FUELING

Cross-country skiers have the highest energy demands found in scientific literature. They can use up to 6,000 calories for daily training. Cross-country skiers, Nordic combined athletes, and biathletes need a lot of energy and carbohydrate. Aim for 8–12 grams per kilogram of body weight per day.

Alpine/downhill skiing, freestyle skiing, and snowboarding use fewer calories overall per session, but adequate calories and carbohydrates are still important. Last season, I was downhill skiing and forgot to eat my regular fueling snacks all morning. By the afternoon, I was so exhausted I fell on the easy green runs. That was my cue to take a break and eat some food!

Skating and hockey athletes usually have more intermittent-type workouts than a cross-country skier, so they use less energy overall. Regardless, they still need adequate calories and carbohydrates. Aim for at least 6 grams of carbs per kilogram of body weight per day.

You may need a vitamin D supplement if you spend a lot of time at high altitude or in cloudy/snowy weather. Check with your doctor to get tested before taking a vitamin D supplement.

Amount	Types of Foods	How to Carry	Tips
Moderate activities (alpine skiing, snowboarding, ice sports, snowshoeing): 45–55 calories/kg body weight per day & 1.2–1.7 g/kg protein per day *Heavy activities:* (ski touring, cross-country skiing, Nordic combined, biathlon): 53–68 calories/kg of body weight per day & 1.4–1.7 g/kg/day of protein Aim for at least 30 g carbs per hour; up to 60–90 g/hour for heavy events like cross-country skiing	Cheese, jerky, nuts, trail mix, gummies, sports gels, energy bars, bread, dried fruit, chocolate, honey, puree pouches (like applesauce), granola, dehydrated or freeze-dried meals, trail mix, canned or pouches of tuna, spam musubi, rice balls, pudding	Close to the body or near armpits if food may freeze Store fuel in easy-access pockets such as the hip pocket on a backpack, front pocket of a jacket, or front pocket of pants.	Package food so you don't have to take your gloves off (easy-to-tear wrappers, water bottles with straws that store in the lid rather than a screw cap, etc.)

AN INTERVIEW WITH MORGAN ARRITOLA, 2010 CROSS-COUNTRY SKIING OLYMPIAN

What are some foods that work well for you to fuel for cross-country skiing?

Nutrition is highly individual and so I would encourage any athlete to work to understand their body's unique needs and also, what do you LIKE?! With cross-country skiing, temperature can be a factor but whether it's summer or winter training, knowing the basic physiological needs of the given workout are important. If you are newer to skiing, ask more seasoned friends or even work with a sport RD. You can also experiment with foods and drinks that taste good, are easy to digest, and fit the bill for your workout and recovery. For example, I hate fruity flavored things so I would avoid bringing something of that flavor because I am also less likely to consume it. I have set myself up to not take the nutrition I know I need. Instead, pack a few options ranging from gels to real food. Lastly, keep it simple. The waters of nutrition can be easily muddied so avoid any "quick fix" or claim that a product will have magical properties. Sometimes a Coke and a cookie does the trick just as well, or better, than an expensive gel product.

Are there any foods that you've found that are easy to carry, don't freeze, easy to eat while on the go, etc?

Sometimes you are in very, very cold temps skiing so again, it depends. I have often used an insulated water bottle and brought hot chocolate or a hot protein mix for during or after cold workouts. At some point, most things freeze, and so maybe you keep a protein bar in an inner pocket, close to your core. Another strategy is to plan training around places that may have a ski hut or village bakery where you can snag something warm and get a break from the snow. Again, you really have to know your goal of the workout and how you maximize the adaptations that can occur from that workout. Lastly, don't aim for perfection. Just think about being consistent over time, and if you have a workout that is longer than expected and maybe you didn't bring food, that's okay! You learned something and the workout is not null just because of the unplanned circumstance.

Do you have a recommendation for how often to eat and drink if you are training a long time (like several hours)?

For me, I preferred real food. I looked forward to eating, which is important because sometimes your body doesn't really want to eat, even though you need it, and tricking your mind into eating can be a good strategy. It can also be easier to eat whole, real food on longer workouts as the intensity is often much lower. Know yourself, what you need, and have a trusted team you can always chat with as those nutritional needs can change over seasons and times of life.

~Morgan Arritola, Former Professional Endurance Athlete, 2010 Olympian, and Licensed Professional Counselor

COMMON METS IN SNOW SPORTS

9.3	Skiing, slalom
4.3	Skiing, downhill, alpine or snowboarding, light effort, active time only
6.3	Skiing, downhill, alpine or snowboarding, moderate effort, general, active time only
8.0	Skiing, downhill, alpine or snowboarding, vigorous effort, active time only
7.3	Skiing, Alpine skiing high-intensity training
5.3	Snowshoeing, moderate effort
10.0	Snowshoeing, vigorous effort
7.0	Skating, ice, general
8.5	Skiing, cross country, 4.0–4.9 mph, moderate speed and effort, general
14.0	Skiing, cross country, elite skier, >8.0–11.9 mph, racing
9.5	Skiing, cross-country skiing high-intensity training
15.5	Skiing, cross country, hard snow, uphill, maximum, snow mountaineering

HIKING

An experienced 62-year-old hiker set out to hike the Pacific Crest Trail. A 2,873-mile journey from the US-Mexican border all the way to the US-Canadian border, this is no small physical feat. Hikers need to coordinate their supplies and food to be brought in to towns along the way. Careful planning is crucial to complete the hike safely.

The woman was selected by researchers to be monitored along her journey. The researchers were curious about how much energy she used each day on the hike. She was expending—or "burning"—an average of 2,634 calories per day, but only eating an average of 1,285 calories per day. This led to weight loss and fatigue, and she was unable to finish her journey.

This woman is not alone in her under-fueling. A research study of twenty-eight men showed their daily energy demands were on average 4,560 calories, but they only brought with them 2,777 calories of fuel per day.

If you don't eat enough food, your body can start breaking down lean tissue for energy. This means muscles and yes, even organ function can be compromised.

Many thru-hikers experience issues such as weight loss, fatigue, poor sleep, poor recovery, and more. And many of these issues could be alleviated or avoided with adequate calories and hydration.

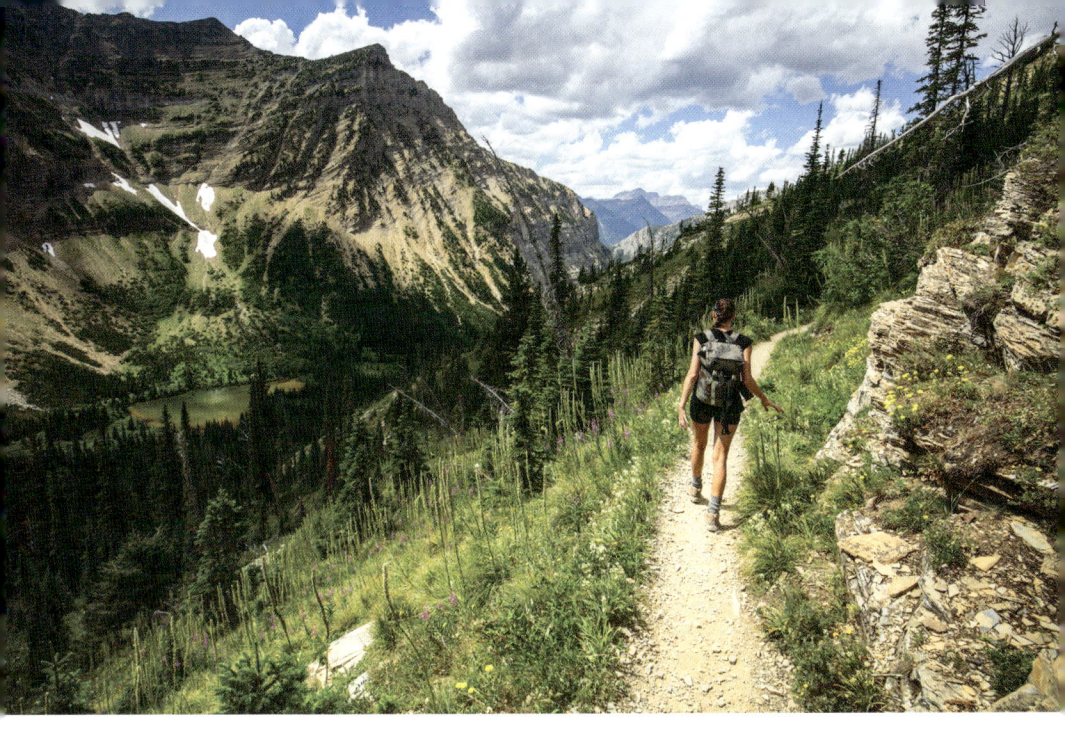

Hikers need to prepare and carry gear for many variables. Depending on the length of the hike, you may have a light day pack, or you may be hiking for several days, weeks, or even months. In any scenario, fueling and hydration are crucial, and being able to carry as little weight as possible is key.

Hikers can face a lot of challenges, including:

- Carrying water if there is no reliable water source on the trail
- Carrying cooking fuel and cooking supplies
- Extreme weather and altitude conditions, which sap energy
- Rugged terrain, which demands more energy to navigate
- Keeping food and supplies sanitary
- Managing gut issues and human waste
- Accumulated stressors on the body from hiking back-to-back days with no recovery time
- Keeping food safe from insects and wildlife
- Loss of appetite at high elevation

Depending on the length of the hike, terrain, weather conditions, and how much gear you need, hikers' nutritional needs can vary a lot. There are also many different types of hiking.

DAY HIKES

Hydration

A good rule of thumb is to start with 8 ounces of water per hour, and then drink more if you have a high sweat rate or the conditions are extreme (i.e., high altitude, heat, or humidity). Depending on your own sweat rate, sodium losses in sweat, and the conditions of the hike, you may or may not need electrolytes. See Chapter 1 for more information on hydration.

Drink regularly to avoid dehydration. Watch your urine color—it should be light yellow. If it is too dark or concentrated, drink more fluids.

Fueling

Fueling needs also vary depending on the terrain, elevation, and your own body. Energy needs are effected by gender, height, weight, age, and level of conditioning.

Aim for at least 30 grams of carbohydrate per hour. Layer in other foods such as trail mix and sandwiches as needed to help you feel full and get a variety of nutrients. Keeping simple carbohydrate snacks accessible can encourage regular fueling. Instead of having to stop and grab food from the back of your pack, keep it in your front pants pockets or the hip pouch of your pack, if you have one.

LONGER HIKES (BACKPACKING/THRU-HIKING/MOUNTAINEERING)

Hydration

Similar to day hikes, aim for regular drinking at regular intervals when possible. Plan your route so that you are by a water source, or calculate your water needs (including cooking and sanitation) so that you can carry enough.

Longer hikes pose a special risk to becoming dehydrated. A day hiker returns to civilization at the end of the day, where rehydrating is often easy to access. A multiday hiker may not be able to fully recover from day to day if they get behind on their hydration needs.

Electrolytes can help retain water in the right spaces and correct amounts in your body. Know beforehand if you are a salty sweater and plan on sodium replacement. This can be done through electrolyte products, adding salt to food, and eating salty foods such as pretzels and salted nuts. Many dehydrated backpacking meals also contain a lot of sodium to help you reach your goals. You may not need to bring electrolytes if you are getting enough sodium from foods. This will save room and weight in your pack.

> **WATER PURIFICATION SYSTEMS**
>
> There are a lot of options for water purification on the market. Do your research and choose one that fits your needs and preferences. Here are a few options:
>
> *Straw style*: This is lightweight and convenient, but doesn't filter water into a bottle or bladder, meaning you don't have a reserve to carry with you. Some products have straws incorporated into a bottle, making it easier to carry some water with you.
>
> *Pump filter*: This can pump water into a bottle or bladder, and has a high rate of pumping, meaning you can pump water pretty fast into whatever container you are using.
>
> *Gravity filter*: These work by filling a bladder with water, then letting it hang while the clean water is filtered down through a tube into your water bottle. This can be nice for group hiking, but there is some wait time. And it's not ideal if you are hiking somewhere without trees or other natural features on which to hang the bladder.
>
> *UV or tablet treatment*: These are tablets you can add to water, but the wait time for it to be safe to drink is sometimes up to 4 hours, meaning it may be impractical for many hikers.
>
> *Squeeze filters*: Popular with thru-hikers because they are lightweight and filter fast. Fill the bottle from a stream, screw the lid on, and drink through the filter.

Aim for 8–16 ounces of fluid per hour and 200–600+ milligrams of sodium per hour.

Fueling

Author's note: Information in this section was kindly provided by Aaron Owens Mayhew, MS, RDN. She has extensive experience with meal planning for thru-hiking. She owns her business, Backcountry Foodie, LLC, where she works with hikers to customize nutrition plans. Her website, backcountryfoodie.com, has lots of resources and free calculators to estimate your food needs on the trail.

General tips: Aim for 30–60 grams of carbohydrate per hour. Snack every 60–90 minutes to keep well fueled throughout the hike and avoid bonking/hitting the wall.

A good rule of thumb is to aim for 5–10 grams/kilogram/day of carbs. Try to get fruits, vegetables, whole grains, beans, and lentils. These complex carbohydrates can offer sustained energy and promote blood sugar stability.

Pack enough food! It is a common mistake to not pack enough. The more strenuous the hike is, the more calories, carbohydrate, and protein you will need.

Nutrient-dense food ideas: Pack foods that provide carbs, protein, and fat in each bite. For example, choose dehydrated quinoa over instant white rice. Choose hummus over a tuna packet. Prepare a homemade oatmeal recipe with oats, nuts, milk powder, and dried fruit instead of just an instant packet of oatmeal. By doing this, the total weight of the food will be less because each bite provides more bang for the buck.

My go-to lunch is hummus because this contains carbs, protein, and fat in a single food. Hikers tend to pack tortillas, tuna, and mayo, but this is three large items compared to one small dish.

Some other nutrient-dense food ideas include:

- Quinoa
- Couscous
- Dehydrated beans, chickpeas, and lentils
- Buckwheat—much higher protein than oats and rehydrates great!
- Hummus mix
- Dairy and non-dairy milk powders—soy, cashew, almond milk powders
- Nut butter powders—peanut, almond, cashew
- Nuts and seeds
- Nut butter
- Nut flours—almond flour is great to thicken smoothies, which adds more nutrition than ground oats. It's also great for coating energy bites so they're less sticky.
- Chia seeds
- Carnation Instant Breakfast
- Egg white powder—an awesome way to add protein without adding weight, doesn't alter the flavor or consistency of the meal
- Whole egg powder—makes great scrambled eggs! See Chapter 7 for the Bacon & Egg Oats recipe using this product.
- Tofu—dehydrates and rehydrates really well. (Freeze it first.) This ingredient weighs next to nothing and adds protein.
- Freeze-dried chicken and beef
- Texturized vegetable protein—mixes great with taco seasoning to make trail tacos
- Freeze-dried fruit—grind it up into a powder using a coffee/spice grinder and add to great smoothies. Very lightweight.

- Baby yogurt melts—A great way to add nutrition to meals without adding weight. Grind it up, just add water, and you have yogurt like you would at home. Yogurt parfait, smoothies, adds creaminess to meals, etc.
- Cold cereal—It's one of the easiest meals to pack. Favorite cold cereal, milk powder, nuts, dried fruit, coconut, chia seeds, whatever fits your fancy. See Chapter 7 for a favorite cold cereal recipe.
- Oil—carry in a small Nalgene bottle

Some other tips from Aaron Owens Mayhew:

- Eat quality food: You will feel better and recover better with whole foods and quality ingredients. Eating low–nutrient-density food is not a good way to support your body when it is under a tremendous load of stress from thru-hiking.
- Many hikers want to carry a lighter pack, so they go into a calorie deficit while hiking, then binge on burgers and beer when they are in town. This is not ideal. If you fuel your hikes adequately as you go, you will feel better and recover better. Find some fresh fruits and vegetables while you're in town to replenish your body.
- Consider adding a multivitamin to your daily routine if you are hiking for months. The dehydration process used to produce backpacking meals can deplete 50–90 percent of water-soluble vitamins.

Sustained-Energy Snacks with 30 Grams of Complex Carbs

Complex carbohydrates provide sustained energy as well as protein, fiber, vitamins, and minerals.

Food	Serving	Carbohydrates (grams)
Apricots, dried	6 apricots	30
Beet chips	2 ounces	32
Brownie batter hummus	1 recipe	39
Classic trail mix	½ cup	24–40
Fritos®	2 ounces	32
Nature's Bakery® fig bar	1 package	38
Peanut butter pretzels	1 ounce	28
Pretzel crisps	1 ounce	24
Walnuts, plain	¾ cup	33

Snack ideas supplied by backcountryfoodie.com

Sample Meal Plan

Note: Every hiker should plan differently based on how their hike will look. Miles per day, time on your feet, speed, height, weight, age, gender, and body composition all play a role in calorie needs. This meal plan is simply a sample of what someone may eat in a day. Your own needs will vary.

Meal	Food	Nutrition Goal
Breakfast 6–7 a.m.	Meal replacement shake, cold cereal, bar	500 calories, 60 g carbs, 20 g protein
Snack 8 a.m.	Trail mix	250 calories, 30 g carbs, 5 g protein
Second breakfast 9 a.m.	Bar with nut butter, oats	600 calories, 60 g carbs, 20 g protein
Snacks 10 a.m.–12 p.m.	Dried fruit, cheese, nuts	500 calories, 60 g carbs, 10 g protein
Lunch 1 p.m.	Loaded baked potato soup (see recipe in Chapter 7), bar	600 calories, 60 g carbs, 20 g protein
Snacks 2–6 pm	Jerky, trail mix, cheese, dried fruit, nut butter	500 calories, 60 g carbs, 10 g protein
Dinner 7 p.m.	Chocolate peanut butter shake (see recipe Chapter 7)	700 calories, 60 g carbs, 20 g protein
Bedtime snack	Meal replacement bar	500 calories, 60 g carbs, 20 g protein

4,150-calorie meal plan

Important Notes

Some reports of scurvy, or vitamin C deficiency, have occurred in thru-hikers. This is because vitamin C is destroyed by heat and the dehydration process, so cooking your food on the trail will not provide any vitamin C in your diet. Hikers often have to eat food that has been cooked, dehydrated, or processed in some way, leaving their food void of vitamin C. To prevent scurvy, try freeze-dried foods that are high in vitamin C, such as strawberries, tomatoes, peppers, and spinach. You can also eat fresh fruits and vegetables when you stop in towns. And foraged greens like dandelions, rose hips, and miner's lettuce can be a safe source of vitamin C.

COMMON METS IN HIKING

7.8 Backpacking, hiking with a daypack
3.8 Hiking slowly or ambling through fields and hillsides, no load
5.3 Hiking or walking at a normal pace through fields and hillsides
7.0 Backpacking
5.3 Climbing hills, no load, 1 to 5 percent grade, moderate-to-brisk pace
8.8 Climbing hills, no load, 11 to 20 percent grade, slow-to-moderate pace
7.5 Climbing hills, 21- to 40-pound load, 3 to 10 percent grade, moderate-to-brisk pace

TRAIL RUNNING

This section will include anything that may apply to trail running, from shorter distances like 5K to ultramarathons. People who do obstacle course races and triathlons can also apply this information to their events.

Trail runners face conditions that pose a challenge to getting proper fueling and hydration. You may have to consider:

- Challenging terrain, often with elevation gain throughout the course
- Many courses take place at high elevation.
- Uneven trail surface means more energy expenditure, as well as need for increased concentration and coordination.
- Self-supported races mean you carry your food, water, and supplies. This additional weight causes extra energy expenditure.
- Extremes in weather, such as wind, heat, cold, or humidity
- The need for rapid recovery in multiday events
- Regulating body temperature in extreme conditions
- Difficulty fueling while holding hiking poles

HYDRATION

Tips to manage hydration on race day:

- Start out well hydrated.
- Fuel early and often, within the first 20–30 minutes.
- Avoid large amounts of fluid at once. Aim for smaller, more frequent drinking to allow your digestion time to absorb.

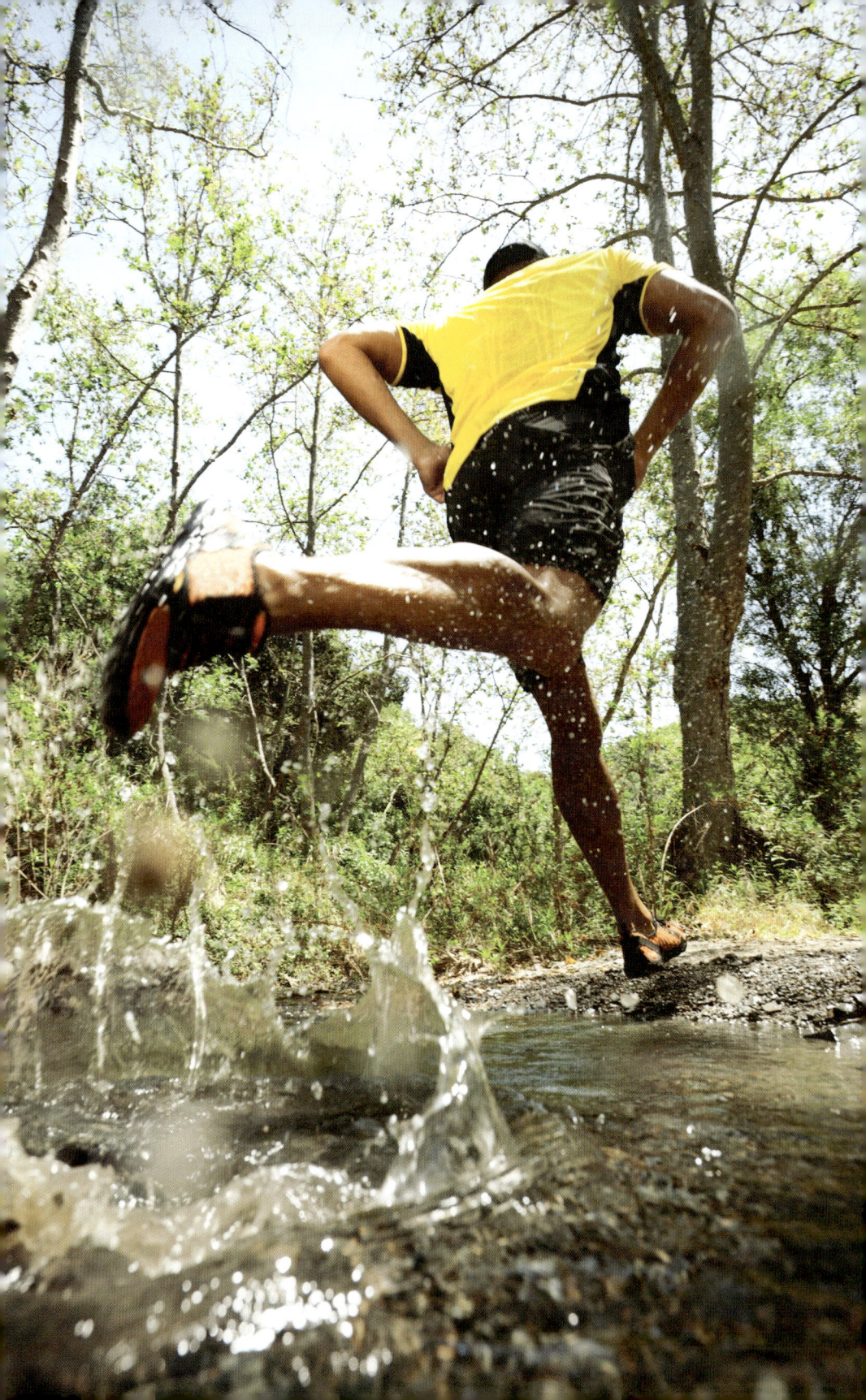

- Add sodium as needed, usually 200–600 milligrams per hour depending on your sweat rate and sodium losses.
- Test your sweat rate during training runs to understand how much fluid per hour you need; practice drinking during training runs.
- Monitor your urine output and color during the race. If you are urinating very infrequently or it is very dark or concentrated, drink more and seek medical attention.

Current guidelines recommend 15–25 ounces of fluid per hour. Pay attention to symptoms of dehydration. For severe sweat losses or prolonged events (lasting several hours), you can replace fluid beyond what you lost. Try to get around 150 percent of your sweat losses in the form of fluids with sodium. This helps replace lost fluid better than water alone.

FUELING

Research from ultramarathon events shows runners used between 3,831 and 4,999 calories per day during a 225 km 5-day event. Another event that was 305 km over 8 days showed energy expenditure between 4,764 and 5,654 calories per day. In a 24-hour trail ultramarathon, runners use up to 18,000 calories.

The average seems to be around 550 calories per hour of race time. Clearly, ultramarathons are a metabolically expensive endeavor. If you do not fuel properly, you could put yourself in danger of a medical emergency, a Did Not Finish, or a very poor experience. Under-fueling can lead to a host of negative health outcomes. For more on this, read about relative energy deficiency in sport in Chapter 6.

Fueling for this event starts way before the event, with two key components:

- Training with fuel and fluids
- Carbohydrate loading 2 to 3 days before the event

TRAINING WITH FUEL AND FLUIDS

It's crucial to fuel your training and test out your gastrointestinal tolerance to certain foods and fluids during these training runs. Practice which foods and fluids you will bring with you, and how often you will eat them in what amounts.

Aim for 150–400 calories per hour, 5–10 grams of protein per hour, and 30–50 grams of carbs per hour. Many people need more than this, up to 80+ grams per hour. This will help with managing blood sugar levels, provide your muscles with fuel, and provide glucose as fuel for your brain.

While this is the goal, research shows that ultrarunners often consume much less, closer to 20–40 grams per hour. Some also consume more, up to 100 grams per hour. Try experimenting during training runs to see what works for you. The more carbohydrate you can tolerate, the better your performance can be. Your gut can be trained! If you start out only being able to take in about 20 grams of carbs per hour, give it time. Slowly increase your intake to 30 and then 40 or more over the course of a few weeks during your training block. Try different types of foods and fluids to see what works best for you. For a list of simple carbs that are easy to eat while exercising, see Chapter 1.

Keep in mind that ultrarunners don't need to rely on only carbohydrate for their fueling needs. Since ultrarunning is often at a low-to-moderate intensity, many runners can tolerate other foods such as trail mix, sandwiches, and protein bars. This can all help you meet your fueling goals.

Taste fatigue is a real thing! It may feel hard to choke down one more gel after being on the course for hours. Consider bringing a mix of tastes and textures to help you stay interested in regularly fueling.

While it may be impossible to match your calorie intake to your calorie output, the closer you can match both energy and carbohydrate needs, the better performance you can have. As long as your gastrointestinal system can handle it, try to fuel as optimally as possible.

During training, energy needs per day need to match expenditure. To understand how many calories you need to eat, you can use your fitness watch to get you in the ballpark. However, these aren't always accurate, but at least it is a starting point. For example, if you go on a 15-mile training run and your device tells you that you've burned 3,500 calories that day, try to eat 3,500 calories throughout the day. You may need more or less than what your device thinks, which you can tailor according to your own outcomes:

- Is your weight remaining stable during training? If so, you are fueling adequately.
- Do you have signs of under-fueling, such as fatigue, poor recovery, and poor training adaptations? If so, you likely need to eat more.

- Aim for 5–8 grams per kilogram per day of carbohydrate during low to moderate training, and 10–12 grams per day during intense or long training or for ultrarunning.

You can also revisit Chapter 1 to understand how to calculate your energy needs, use METS to determine energy expenditure during a training run, or meet with a sports dietitian for a more precise and personalized plan.

Ultrarunner carbohydrate needs are high, at around 8–12 grams per kilogram per day. Protein needs are around 1.6–1.8 grams per kilogram per day. Day-to-day training needs for shorter distances may require a bit less—around 1.2–1.6 grams/kilogram protein daily and 5–8 grams/kilogram of carbs daily.

Carbohydrate Loading

This should happen 2 to 3 days before the event. Carb loading is not just eating a spaghetti dinner the night before. It is careful planning days prior. It's also wise to test out carb loading during your training cycle. Try it a few days before a very long run (2+ hours) to test for tolerance before race day.

The purpose of carb loading is to increase your glycogen stores (this is the storage form of sugar in your muscles and liver). Glycogen is the fuel for muscle contraction. There is ample research on carbohydrate loading. It can help you prevent bonking and go longer until exhaustion, and also increase race pace.

To carb load correctly, you need to eat 12 grams per kilogram of carbs per day for 2 to 3 days. This will feel like a lot of carbs! Try to focus on food sources of carbohydrate that are lower in fiber. This enables you to eat more without feeling too full, and also allows for your bowels to not have as much stool in them on the day of the race. Many people eat things like an entire pack of white bagels in one day when they are carb loading.

If you find yourself struggling to get enough food, this may be due to a decreased appetite. It is common for hunger cues to go away with intense endurance training. This does not mean you don't need to eat! Since your hunger cues may not be reliable, you have to rely on your nutrition knowledge. Remember how crucial it is to fuel properly, and eat even when you don't feel like it.

> **SAMPLE CARB LOADING MENU FOR SOMEONE AROUND 110–120 POUNDS**
>
> *Breakfast:*
> 1 cup Corn Flakes
> 8 oz 1 percent milk
> 1 banana
>
> *Snack:*
> 6 oz yogurt with fruit
>
> *Lunch:*
> Turkey sandwich on a hoagie roll, lettuce, tomato
> 1 c grapes
> 2 oz pretzels
>
> *Snack:*
> 2 sheets graham crackers
> 8 oz 1 percent milk
>
> *Dinner:*
> 4 c pasta, cooked
> 1 c marinara sauce
> 3 oz ground beef, cooked
> 1 sweet potato
> 16 oz Gatorade
>
> *Snack:*
> 1 blueberry muffin
> 8 oz orange juice
>
> Total: 3,147 calories, 488 grams carbohydrate, 125 grams protein

Tips to manage low hunger:

- Drink your calories. Fluids are often easier to stomach than solid food. Try smoothies, protein shakes, milk, chocolate milk, and hearty soups.
- Eat lower-fiber foods if higher fiber makes you feel too full too fast. Swap out whole grain bread for white bread, white bagels, or rolls. Use white rice instead of quinoa. Have one vegetable side dish instead of a giant salad as your main course.
- Eat early and often. Eat every 1 to 2 hours. Don't delay or skip breakfast. Set a timer on your phone or watch to remind you to eat or drink something with calories.
- Drink or eat something within an hour of working out.

- Add extra calories to foods you already eat, like adding canola oil to a smoothie, using butter to sauté vegetables, switching to full fat dairy products, etc.

Options to carry food and fluids:

- Single-use fuel such as gels or pouches
- Reusable soft silicone flasks filled with your fuel of choice
- Small pack with a water bladder and drinking hose
- Handheld water bottle
- Carry both plain water and fluid with electrolytes (and/or carbohydrate depending on personal preference)
- Small backpack
- Running vest with water bottle and fuel pockets
- Running belt
- Built-in pockets in clothing

Tips to manage gastrointestinal issues:

- Avoid aspirin, acetaminophen, naproxen, and ibuprofen when possible. These are known to cause stomach upset.
- Train with fuel and fluids to train your gut to tolerate them on race day.
- Use a variety of carbohydrate sources. Certain carbohydrate molecules have a limit to how much can be absorbed at one time in your intestine. Mixing your carbohydrate sources to include a variety of sugars, such as glucose and fructose, increases your intestine's ability to absorb them.
- Include sodium, as this is a key mineral involved with carbohydrate absorption. It also is the main electrolyte lost in sweat.
- Include electrolytes in your fluids to enable them to be absorbed and help your body maintain proper fluid balance.
- Avoid common triggers like caffeine, chocolate, peppermint, and citrus if these bother your stomach.
- Avoid high-fiber foods a few days before the race.
- Allow yourself time on race day morning to have a bowel movement.
- Avoid alcohol and marijuana products if these cause gastrointestinal issues for you.

Be sure you understand the nature of the race so you can plan accordingly:

- Know if the race organizers are providing any fuel or fluids.
- Know where the support stations are located on the course, how far apart they are, and what they offer.
- Know if you are required to bring your own food and supplies.
- Know if there is a weight limit to your pack.

Food ideas for ultramarathon or long trail events at low- to mid-intensity:

- Salted mashed potatoes in silicone flask
- Pudding in silicone flask
- Pickles
- Trail mix
- Granola bars
- Dried fruit
- Sandwiches
- Nut butters
- Muffins
- Jerky
- Sausage sticks
- Cheese sticks
- Cheese-flavored crackers
- Protein bars
- Potato chips
- Flat or carbonated caffeinated soda
- Dates
- Sports drinks
- Sports gels
- Gummies
- Pretzels
- Pastries

SAMPLE RACE DAY FUELING PLAN (YOU MAY NEED MORE OR LESS THAN THIS BASED ON YOUR OWN BODY AND THE RACE CONDITIONS)

Half-day race (2–5 hours)

Breakfast: Cereal, milk, fruit

During race: Every hour 8 oz Gatorade, 2 packs fruit snacks

After race: Fluid with electrolytes, rice, chicken, and salad

Night snack: Protein shake, fruit

Full-day race (8+ hours)

Pre-race breakfast: Oatmeal, milk, fruit

During race:

1st hour: 2 packs fruit snacks, 8 oz Gatorade

2nd hour: 1 oz pretzels, 8 oz Gatorade

3rd hour: Trail mix, 8 oz water

4th hour: 2 gels, 8 oz water

5th hour: Peanut butter and jelly sandwich, 8 oz Gatorade

6th hour: 2 packs fruit snacks, 8 oz water

7th hour: 2 Rice Krispie treats, 8 oz Gatorade

8th hour: 2 gels, 8 oz water

After race: Hamburger, smoothie, Gatorade

Night snack: Chocolate milk, turkey sandwich

COMMON METS IN TRAIL RUNNING

9.3	Running, cross country
10.3	Running uphill, 4.5 mph, 5 percent incline
17.5	Running uphill, 5.0 to 5.9 mph, 15 percent incline
13.5	Running uphill, 1.2 to 1.39 mph, 30 to 40 percent incline
5.8	Running downhill, 5.0 to 5.9 mph, -10 percent to -15 percent
9.3	Running downhill, 6.0 to 7.9 mph, -3 percent to -9 percent

CLIMBING

This section covers fueling for most types of climbing, including sport, ice, trad, top rope, bouldering, and via ferrata. Since speed climbing is an indoor sport, it will not be covered in-depth in this section. Nutrition demands for day-to-day training are similar to overall climbing nutrition needs.

HYDRATION

You've read about hydration in Chapter 1, and those principles also apply here. Hydration is important for sports performance, and in the context of climbing it is even more important. Climbing demands a sharp mind to keep you and your partner safe at the crag. Dehydration can compromise mental acuity. One missed knot or safety check could spell disaster.

A general rule of thumb for climbing is to drink about 8 ounces per hour. As you've learned from other parts of this book, your hydration strategy depends on a variety of factors, such as individual sweat rate, individual sodium losses in sweat, altitude, and environmental conditions (heat, humidity, cold, wind, etc.).

To ensure good hydration, you can watch your urine color. If it is light yellow, you are doing great. If it is dark or concentrated, or you urinate infrequently, drink more. Aim to drink enough to avoid greater than 2 percent loss of your body weight. See Chapter 1 for more on how to weigh yourself to measure your sweat rate.

FUELING

Climbers are notoriously under-fueled. There are several studies at the time of this writing that show climbers do not eat enough to match their training load.

Eating enough can help support climbing performance and overall health. For more about the risks of under-fueling, see Chapter 6.

Climbing on average burns about 10–11 calories per minute of active climbing. Although the actual expenditure varies from person to person and depends on the nature of the climbing, most climbers use about 250–400 calories per hour during active climbing sessions.

Carbohydrate needs are 3 to 5 grams per kilogram per day, and about 30–60 grams per hour. A climber who also ends up hiking long distances to get to and from the crag will need more carbohydrate, around 6–8 grams per kilogram per day total, and 30–60 grams per hour during active hiking and climbing sessions. See Chapter 1 for a list of ideas of simple carbs to eat while climbing.

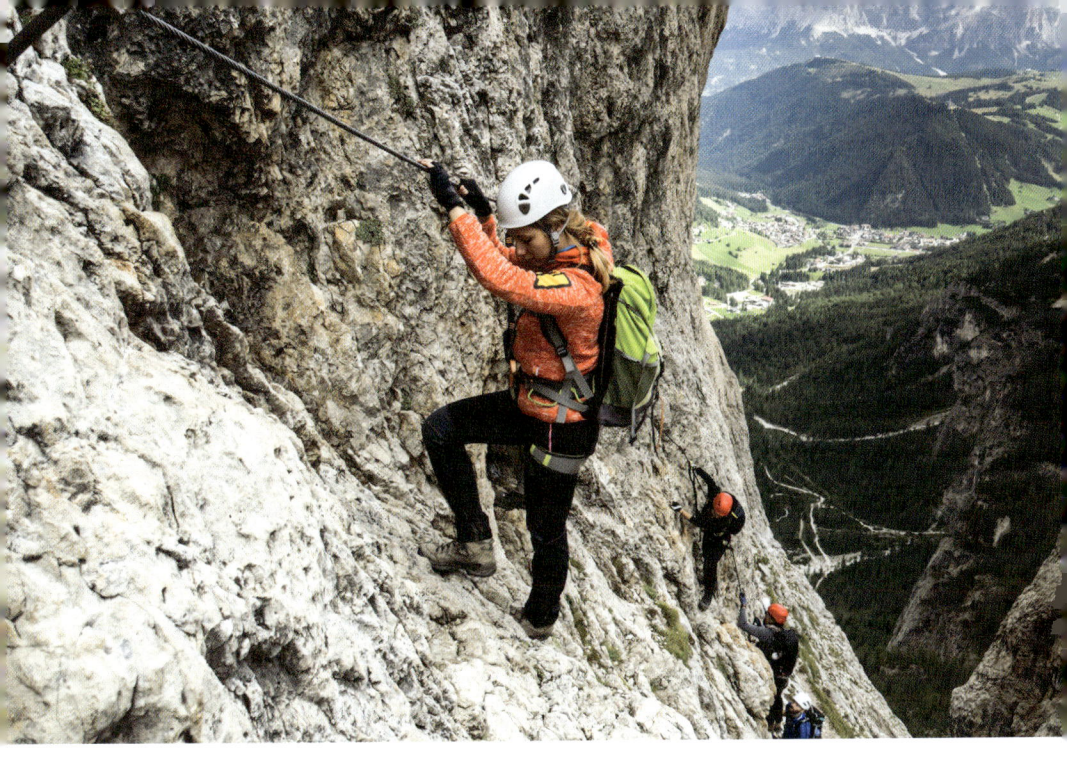

Climbers need around 1.4–1.8 grams per kilogram of protein per day. Up to 2.0 grams per kilogram is appropriate if they are in a strength or power endurance training phase.

> **A MENU FOR A DAY AT THE CRAG MIGHT LOOK LIKE THIS:**
>
> Breakfast at home: Oatmeal with berries, nuts, and milk, 2 eggs
>
> Hike to crag: 1 oz pretzels and 8 oz water
>
> Climb 9 a.m.–12 p.m.: Dried fruit, graham crackers, and fruit snacks at 30-60 grams per hour plus water or sports drink 8 oz per hour
>
> Lunch: Peanut butter and jelly sandwich, apple, shelf-stable chocolate milk, and trail mix
>
> Climb 1 p.m.–5 p.m.: Banana, gummies, and white bagel at 30-60 grams per hour plus water or sports drink 8 oz per hour
>
> Hike back from crag: Energy bar, sports drink
>
> Dinner at home: Fish tacos with salad, smoothie, and a side of black beans

SAMPLE COMP-DAY MENU WITH MULTIPLE ROUNDS

Event	Time	Time Eaten	Food
Breakfast	8 a.m.	Prior to event	Steel cut oats with walnuts, berries, and milk. Orange juice as a beverage.
Round 1 climbing	10 a.m.	After event	Pretzels and sports drink
Round 2 climbing	12 p.m.	After event	Peanut butter and jam sandwich on white bread with apple slices. Chocolate milk as a beverage.
Round 3 climbing (isolation)	3 p.m.	Eat/drink as needed in isolation	Sports gummies and sports drink
Round 4 climbing	5 p.m.	Prior to event as required	Raisins and sports drink
Dinner	7 p.m.	After event	Quinoa bowl with black beans, salsa, cheese, avocado, and ground beef with a fruit and yogurt smoothie

Source: Michael, M. K., O. C. Witard, L. Joubert, and R. Taiar. "Physiological Demands and Nutritional Considerations for Olympic-Style Competitive Rock Climbing," *Cogent Medicine* 6, no. 1 (2019).

The focus before and during climbing is carbohydrates. This is because it fuels the energy systems used in climbing movements. However, if you find that carbohydrates leave you hungry or you need more lasting energy, eat more carbs per hour or layer in some protein, fiber, and fat. While these nutrients do not provide ready energy for climbing, they can help blood sugar levels remain more stable and help contribute to a feeling of fullness. Make carbohydrate the center of your snack, but add protein, fiber, and fat on the side as needed.

This may look like eating some gummies and pretzels, but also adding a nut butter pouch. It could also be eating a large bagel and apple, but adding a pouch of tuna. Experiment with what works for you. You may find that certain foods settle in your stomach better than others. It's hard to climb with a full or upset stomach. Try to avoid too much fiber or fat if you are struggling with this.

Signs you may be under-fueling during a climbing session:

- Weak or shaky hands
- Inability to concentrate or figure out the beta
- Forgetting safety checks
- Breakthrough hunger
- Lack of motivation
- Lack of power
- Decreased or plateaued endurance
- Easy moves feel hard or impossible

REMEMBERING TO EAT AND DRINK

It's easy to forget to fuel while climbing. An all-day cragging outing can involve a long approach to the crag, lots of gear management, and multi-pitch adventures where gear is heavy; and food and water can be at the bottom of your packing list.

To help you remember to eat and drink, try the following:

- Bring a variety of food that you know you will eat. Taste fatigue is real. Bring both sweet and savory options.
- Add calories to your water by using a sports drink mix if you struggle to eat enough food.
- Time your fueling and hydration within the normal pace of the day. Eat during natural breaks, such as when you switch belayers, when you flake the rope, when you finish a pitch, etc.
- Bring more water than you think you need, especially if you are not climbing near a water source.
- Put a timer on your phone or watch to go off every hour. Eat or drink something when the timer beeps.

COMMON METS IN CLIMBING

8.0	Rock or mountain climbing
8.8	Rock climbing, free boulder
7.3	Rock climbing, ascending rock, high difficulty
10.5	Rock climbing, speed climbing, very difficult
5.8	Rock climbing, ascending or traversing rock, low-to-moderate difficulty
10.5	Rock climbing, treadwall, 4–6 m/min
10.5	Rock climbing, treadwall, 7–10 m/min
5.0	Rock climbing, rappelling

AN INTERVIEW WITH AMITY WARME

Amity Warme has an impressive tick list of Yosemite sends, in addition to being a registered dietitian with a master's in sports nutrition. She is an amazing athlete and thoughtful dietitian. She was kind enough to allow me to interview her. Please enjoy partaking from her wealth of knowledge.

Marisa: How do you prep food for a big wall climb?

Amity: First, I plan out the number of days that we will be on the wall, then account for breakfast, lunch/day snacks, and dinner for each of those days. As I'm packing, I lay out all my meals and snacks and separate them by day. Life on a big wall is already logistically complicated, so the more food prep I can do beforehand, the easier it makes things on the wall. I'll group, bag, and label each day's worth of food so that it is easy to find in the haul bag and portion out when on the wall. There is no way to refrigerate things up there so that means mostly dehydrated or freeze-dried meals for breakfast and dinner and lots of energy bars, trail mix, and other easily portable snack foods that provide both carbs and protein. Additionally, space and weight are at a premium, so maximizing energy density is important.

Marisa: Do you have certain foods you always bring or always avoid? Why?

Amity: Yep! I have found some go-tos that work really well for me. I tend to rely on these things because I know they will provide good energy, help with recovery for back-to-back days, and not cause gastrointestinal distress while on the wall. I'm always trying to dial things in though, and I think my fueling strategy gets better with each big wall mission I do!

Always bring:

- Pre-made oatmeal packs with my favorite fixings
- Dried fruit (my favorite are figs!)
- A salty nut or seed (my favorite are pumpkin seeds!)
- My favorite quick energy bar (EnduroBites)
- Dinner with high protein and carbs

Avoid bringing:

- In my day-to-day life on the ground, I love eating tons of fresh fruits and vegetables, but those things just aren't realistic in a big wall setting. I always crave a crunchy, juicy apple when I'm up there for days on end eating nothing but dried food, so sometimes I'll sneak in one or two, but for the most part fresh produce is what I miss the most up there and am always eager to eat when I get down.

Marisa: Do you have a certain fueling and hydration schedule when climbing? What does a typical day look like on the wall?

Amity: My fueling and hydration schedule is not super rigid when I'm on the wall because it is dictated by the climbing schedule, which can vary quite a bit day to day depending on conditions, which pitches we are trying that day, how many pitches, etc. So, the timing can vary, but generally speaking, a typical day would look like:

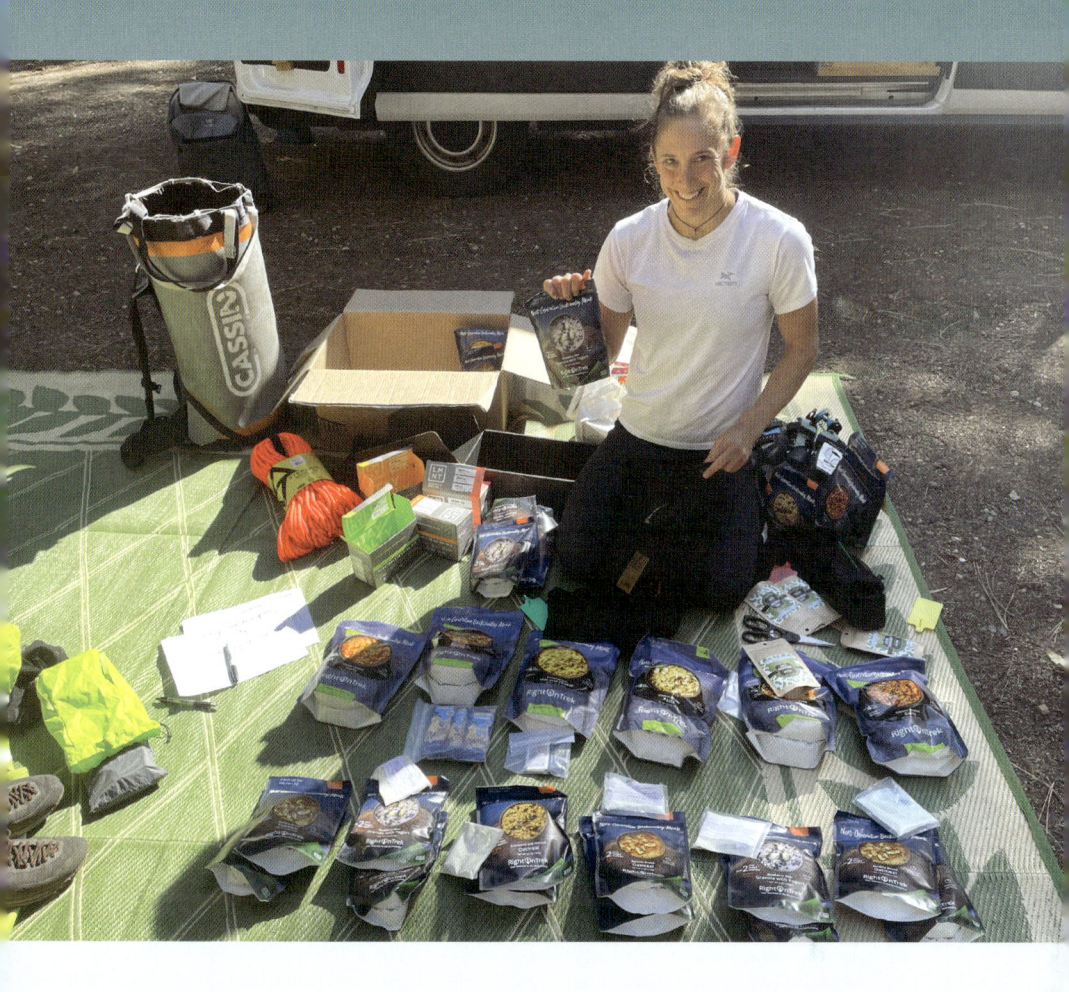

Breakfast: usually pretty early because you tend to wake up with the sun up there

- Oatmeal with protein powder, dried fruit, chia seeds, and cinnamon
- Coffee

Snacking throughout the day: I generally don't eat a full "lunch" because I am on the move pretty much all day and it works better for me to just be really consistent about munching on something between every pitch. A long, involved pitch plus hauling up to a couple hundred pounds of supplies up after you uses a ton of energy, so I try to eat something between every pitch. Some typical options include:

- Bagels
- Bars (EnduroBites, protein bar, RX bars)
- Dried fruit (figs, dates, mango, apricots, etc.)
- Nut butter packets
- Something salty like pretzels or nuts/seeds

(continued)

5 / FUELING YOUR ADVENTURE   **125**

Dinner: I aim to get at least 25 grams of protein and 75–100 grams of carbs to help me refuel and recover in order to perform at a high level again the next day. This could be a homemade combo or one of many prepackaged options.

- RightOnTrek packaged dinners worked really well for me on my most recent climb. The cooking method with this brand makes them easier to digest than many packaged, dehydrated meals, they met my macronutrient criteria that I aim for, and they tasted great. We split four portions between three people to make sure we were all getting enough!

Dessert: a couple bites of chocolate is a tasty way to cap off the evening.

Marisa: How do you know how much food to bring?

Amity: Under-fueling on a big wall climb is one of the biggest mistakes I see people make. You set yourself up for so much more success if you bring enough food. It is super easy to underestimate the amount of food you need when you are up there for multiple days in a row because when you are on the ground packing, it looks like a *ton* of food to haul. The energy expenditure while big wall climbing is extreme though!! Of course, the climbing itself takes a lot of energy, but then you add hauling a couple hundred pounds of gear plus exposure to the elements and additional psychological stress. All this adds up to massive energy expenditure! And each day compounds on the previous day, so if you are rationing food straightaway, you are just setting yourself up to be in a massive calorie deficit that will have a hugely detrimental effect on your performance, attitude, and decision-making skills. My fueling strategies have improved with each big wall I've done, but mostly this just means bringing much more food than I used to!

Marisa: Do you use electrolytes when doing big wall climbing?

Amity: I do use electrolytes! A lot of the time up there I am exposed to the sun and other elements. Plus, I am almost constantly in motion so I end up losing a lot of fluid and electrolytes through sweat.

The typical water allocation is 1 gallon per person per day. This includes enough water for drinking plus cooking breakfasts and dinners. Logistically this is important because of the amount of weight it adds up to. Of course, you are hauling all your water up from the ground with you; so, for example, on my most recent big wall climb, we hauled 175 pounds of water because we were planning for 7–8 days for three people (myself, my climbing partner, and a videographer).

Staying hydrated is super important though, and I think an electrolyte can help maintain proper hydration levels. My favorite to bring on a big wall is LMNT because it contains a high amount of sodium (and other electrolytes) and because the single serve packets are really convenient up there. It's nice to have a little packet versus trying to scoop from a big container when you're on the wall—again, convenience is everything on the wall. I like that LMNT isn't syrupy sweet like some electrolytes are because I get tired of sweet, flavored bars and things while on the wall. LMNT doesn't have the carb content that many sports drinks do, but I make up for that by just eating more carbs throughout the day instead of drinking them.

IMPORTANT NOTES

The climbing community is plagued with stories of disordered eating. This often stems from the idea that climbing ability is dependent on a high strength-to-weight ratio. The problem is, the "weight" part of the "strength-to-weight" ratio is often focused on. Many climbers try to lose weight in order to improve climbing performance. However, this is fraught with risks such as disordered eating, relative energy deficiency in sport, heightened injury risk, and loss of lean muscle mass. Chapter 6 will go into more detail about these risks.

The idea of losing weight to enhance climbing performance is not supported by current evidence. Anthropometrics—or measurable body characteristics like weight, height, and ape index—are not correlated to climbing ability. Instead, focus on other variables such as endurance, finger strength, overall strength, technical skills, and flexibility. An under-fueled climber is an under-performing climber. Falling into the trap of losing weight to send your project will not set you up for success.

Below is a chart summarizing the current evidence on climbing ability and anthropometrics. Note that most evidence points toward body weight and body composition being largely irrelevant to climbing ability. Hours of training per week, years of experience, and other more controllable variables such as strength and flexibility are more likely to reward you with improved climbing than weight loss.

Study	Summary of Findings
Grønahug (2018)	BMI, climbing ability, and injuries had no correlation.
Arazi (2017)	Body fat and BMI didn't have an effect on climbing performance.
Laffaye (2016)	Only 4% of climbing ability is due to anthropometrics.
Mermier (2000)	Only 1.8% of climbing ability is due to anthropometrics.
Ozimek (2017)	Elite climbers had lower body weight and body fat, better finger strength, and better arm endurance.
Laval (2019)	Weight was not correlated with climbing ability. Flexibility, shoulder strength, endurance, and finger strength were.
Saul (2019)	BMI is not associated with higher climbing ability. Bent arm hangs, hand grip strength, endurance, and forearm flexors were.

(continued)

Study	Summary of Findings
Michael (2019)	BMI and weight are not associated with climbing ability. Years climbing and hours per week training were.
Giles (2020)	Years climbing, training hours per week, finger strength, forearm volume, power slap; body fat was lower in elite vs. advanced.
Vereide (2022)	No significant difference in body mass or fat mass between intermediate and elite climbers or between advanced and elite climbers. "It cannot be concluded that this metric has a meaningful impact on performance among climbers." "Training and climbing experience may be crucial factors for improving climbing performance."

BIKING

This section can apply to many different types of biking, including recreational adventures, gravel biking, mountain biking, and formal races such as downhill, cross-country, and stage racing. Biking has similar nutrition and hydration needs as trail running. The demands are high and fueling early and often is key to success, especially if it is a very long race, such as 24-hour races or 100-mile races. If you're a mountain biker heading out for a half-day or full-day ride, fueling and hydration are still very important.

Off-road biking has a higher energy demand than road cycling, and most bikers are working at close to their maximum heart rate and VO_2 max for the duration of the ride.

HYDRATION

Hydration needs can vary widely based on your own sweat rate, altitude, intensity of the ride, and temperature. See Chapter 1 for more information on hydration and sweat rate. Aim for at least 8–16 ounces per hour of fluids.

Aim to replace your lost fluids after your ride. Electrolytes can be useful, especially if you are a salty sweater or notice fatigue or headaches after riding.

Carrying fluids on the bike is usually easy if you have multiple water bottle holders. If you are self-supported and going all day, you can also add a bladder-hose system in a backpack. This is a good option if your route is not near a water source where you could easily refill empty bottles.

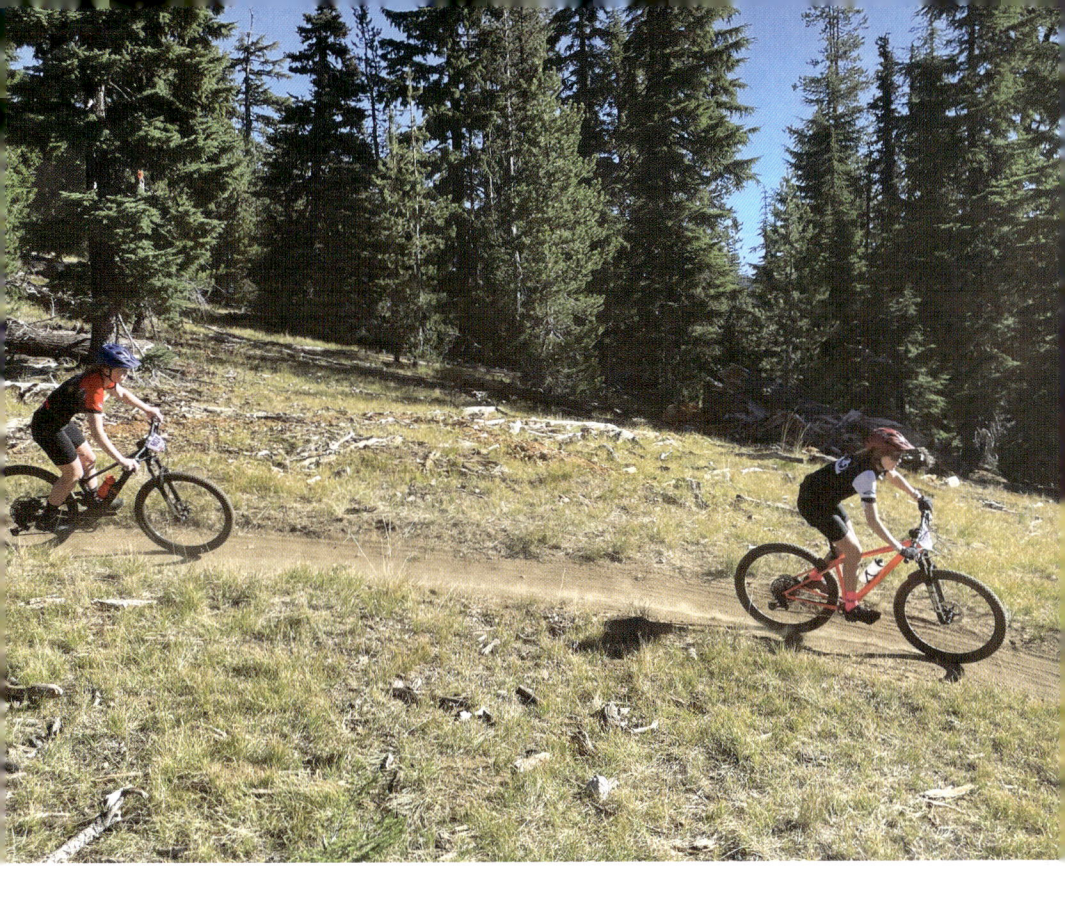

FUELING

As with many other sports, eating simple carbohydrates at regular intervals is important. Aim for at least 30–60 grams per hour of riding. You may need more for long or intense riding. Some pro riders use up to 90–120 grams per hour. If you are going at a lower intensity, other foods can be added if your stomach and gut can tolerate it. More complex foods that contain fat, fiber, and protein can help you feel fuller longer for all-day rides. Sandwiches or wraps, rice balls, trail mix, jerky, nut butter, or granola bars are all easy, portable choices.

COMMON METS IN MOUNTAIN BIKING

- 14.0 Bicycling, mountain, uphill, vigorous
- 16.0 Bicycling, mountain, competitive racing
- 8.5   Bicycling, BMX
- 8.5   Bicycling, mountain, general
- 5.8   Bicycling, on dirt or farm road, moderate pace

IMPORTANT NOTES

Fueling and hydration can be a real challenge, as it's hard to eat and drink on the bike, especially if the trail is very technical and demands all your concentration (and hands on the handlebars!). Try building in rest and fueling breaks off your bike if this is the case.

If you are in a racing situation where taking a leisurely break off your bike is not an option, start out well fueled and well hydrated. If you are able to drink during the race, use your fluid as both fuel and hydration by utilizing a sports drink with carbohydrate. Practice fueling while riding where it is safe and possible to do so. This might look like unwrapping a bar partway and taping it on your top tube, having gummies in an open plastic bag in your jersey pocket for easy reaching and snacking, or having a bento box accessory mounted on your bike full of simple carbohydrate snacks. Be familiar with the course aid stations, where they are located, and what foods and fluids will be offered so you can plan your strategy correctly.

It isn't necessary to exactly replace all the calories and fluid you are expending on the ride, but it is important to fuel and hydrate regularly. The longer

> **WHAT BIKERS ATE IN A 24-HOUR RACE**
>
> Researchers studied seventy-four mountain bikers competing in a 24-hour race. In the month before the race, 64 percent ate a high-carb diet. The day before the race, 84 percent ate a high-carb diet.
>
> During the race:
>
> 86.5 percent of racers ate bananas
>
> 50 percent ate energy bars
>
> 43 percent ate apples
>
> After the race:
>
> 45 percent ate bread
>
> 34 percent ate rice
>
> 34 percent ate bananas
>
> During the race:
>
> 82 percent drank a sports drink
>
> 54 percent drank Coca-Cola
>
> 72 percent drank water
>
> On average, each racer ate 30.6 times during the 24-hour race!

the course, the more carbohydrate you need per hour. For a shorter course under 2 hours, 30–60 grams per hour should suffice. For longer courses, all-day rides, or 24-hour racing, 60–100 grams per hour is ideal.

If you're a recreational rider, self-supported fueling and hydration is important. Carry more water and food than you think you will need. A variety of foods and tastes (sweet, salty, savory) can help avoid taste fatigue and encourage better fueling. Know the route and if you need to bring water, or if you can bring along a filter and pump water as you go.

WATER SPORTS

My friend asked me if I wanted to do a race with her. "It's a run-swim-run-swim-run-swim race," she said. Um, what? "You have to run in your wetsuit and swim with your shoes on." She then describes the logistics: running to a body of water, swimming across, jumping out, and doing that on repeat. "And you have to seal your food in a little baggie and tuck it into your wetsuit," she adds.

This sounds miserable to me. Even though I didn't want to actually do this race, the sports dietitian side of me was intrigued. How would I plan out a fueling and hydration strategy for this? You have to carry foods, fluids, and all your gear . . . while swimming and running!

Such is the case with many water sports. They pose some unique fueling challenges. There may be tricky logistics, depending on the type of water sport you're doing. For example, open water swimming does not allow an easy way to carry or eat food during the swim, so careful planning is essential to start the swim well fueled and well hydrated, or have a support vehicle alongside the swimmer to offer fuel and hydration as needed for prolonged events.

Paddling sports vary widely in their duration. From a 1-hour chill standup paddleboard float to a vigorous, multiday whitewater rafting trip, your fueling and hydration strategy will need to match the activity.

Surfing often presents more extreme environmental conditions, such as heat and humidity or prolonged exposure to open water.

This section aims to cover all types of water sports. Since they vary so much in their duration, intensity, and movement patterns, we'll go over some general tips to consider for some water sports. You can use the information you learned in Chapters 1 and 2 to customize it for your own needs and sport. If you're doing a new, prolonged, or intense activity it's always wise to consult with a sports dietitian for a personalized plan.

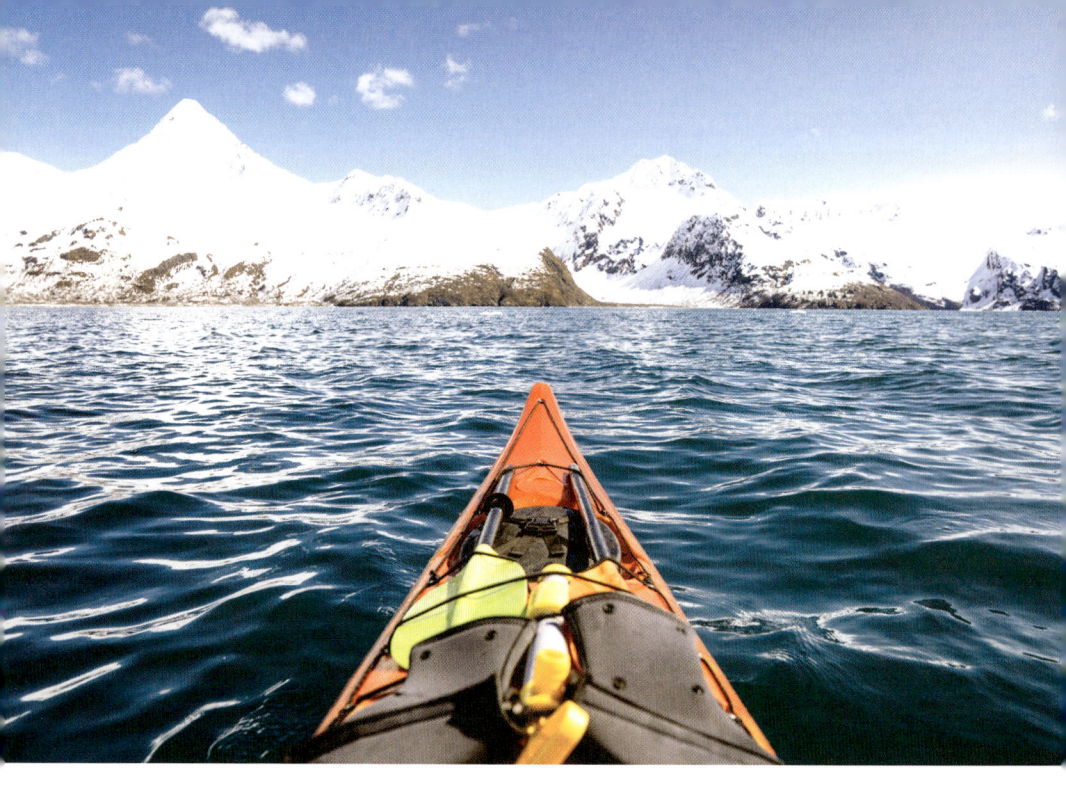

HYDRATION

Hydration needs vary widely based on the sport, the temperature, altitude, and your own sweat rate. Water sports may be harder to hydrate at regular intervals than other sports. A runner or hiker can sip while moving. A cyclist can get water while riding. A skier or climber can sip from a bladder/hose system in a backpack. But for a surfer or swimmer, hydration can be a logistical challenge. Some water sports involve a boat, canoe, kayak, or raft, making an easy way to stash water and food. Depending on your sport, you may have to get creative and purposeful about hydration.

General needs are at least 8 ounces per hour. To understand more about how to tailor your hydration plan to your situation, see Chapter 1 for fluid information and Chapter 3 for special situations (like heat or high altitude).

If you are a swimmer, sweat rates are generally lower in the water than land-based activities, so you may need less fluids per hour than if you were on dry land.

FUELING

General fueling principles apply to water sports! A rule of thumb is to aim for at least 30 grams of carbohydrate per hour of activity. If it is a low-intensity activity such as canoeing across a flat lake, your stomach can probably tolerate most types of foods without issues, such as trail mix, jerky, sandwiches, cheese, or a tuna pouch.

For more intense activities, like open water swimming or surfing, there is no opportunity to fuel while you're doing the activity itself. This means planning before and after will be important. Eat a full meal about 3–4 hours before your activity. This gives your body enough time to digest, but also allows your body some nourishment. Then, within 60 minutes of your activity, have an easy-to-digest, simple carbohydrate snack like a white bagel, pretzels, or gummies. Go swim or surf, and then have a full meal within 2 hours of stopping your activity. This will give your body the nourishment it needs to recover.

Keep in mind that water temperature can impact your body's energy needs. Very cold water—or even moderate temperatures—can often demand higher energy output, as well as challenge your ability to regulate your own body temperature. Hypothermia can result even in water temperatures that are mildly lower than your body temperature if you are in water for a prolonged period.

IMPORTANT NOTES

In open water swim events in warm climates, there have been reports of overheating and hyponatremia (low blood sodium) due to athletes drinking so

---

COMMON METS IN WATER SPORTS

- 13.5 Kayaking, competition
- 4.0 Fishing from a riverbank, standing and walking
- 2.0 Fishing from a boat or canoe, sitting
- 4.0 Canoeing, on camping trip
- 5.0 Kayaking, moderate effort
- 15.5 Rowing
- 6.0 Waterskiing or wakeboarding
- 5.8 Scuba diving, general, moderate effort
- 3.0 Surfing, body or board, general
- 6.5 Stand up paddleboarding, general
- 10.5 Swimming, open water 5K
- 6.0 Swimming, lake, ocean, river
- 5.0 Whitewater rafting, kayaking, or canoeing
- 11.0 Windsurfing or kitesurfing

much that they dilute their blood sodium. Be careful if you are competing in prolonged events like these.

Stashing food in a dry bag can be really helpful for water sports involving a boat, canoe, raft, or kayak. Wet, soggy food is not appealing and possibly not safe to eat if the water was contaminated, putting you at risk of hypoglycemia.

If you're on a multiday water adventure, be sure to eat and drink enough at the end of the day to replenish glycogen stores and rehydrate. This way, you'll be set up for the next day. Back-to-back days of intense sports can deplete the body quickly. Be mindful of how your body is feeling. Eating and drinking enough can help you feel better and be energized for your multiday trip.

Try eating something with carbohydrate when you finish. Aim for 1 gram per kilogram of body weight. So if you weigh 70 kilograms, eat at least 70 grams of carbohydrate within the first 4 hours. Continue eating at regular intervals, every 3–4 hours (except when you are sleeping) to replenish spent glycogen stores. Aim for at least 20–30 grams of protein with each meal as well.

CAMPING

Camping at its core is simply living outdoors. Since it's not a sport, this section will focus more on camping food preparation and ideas. Camping doesn't necessarily require specific fueling or hydration recommendations, although it's smart to be aware of how hydrated you are, and any environmental conditions (altitude, heat, etc.) that would impact how to fuel and hydrate.

FOOD AND CAMPGROUND SAFETY

Camping poses unique challenges with food storage and preparation. Keeping perishable foods cold enough can be an issue, especially for trips longer than a couple of days. Replace your cooler ice often to make sure your food stays at a safe temperature to prevent food poisoning.

Keep food away from wildlife. Don't store it on top of a picnic table or on the ground. Keep it locked in bear lockers if they are available. Otherwise, store it in your vehicle unless the campground forbids it (some bears break into vehicles). Store trash responsibly according to your campground rules. Keep it away from raccoons, rodents, bears, insects, and other creatures.

When prepping, make sure any raw meat or egg doesn't contaminate other foods. Use separate knives and cutting boards, or wash them between uses with hot soapy water. Wash or sanitize all surfaces, including your hands, plates, and utensils after they come in contact with raw meat or eggs. Store raw meat and eggs in sealed containers separate from the rest of the items in your cooler. Don't leave perishable food out for more than 2 hours.

Cook meats to an internal temperature of 165 degrees. Throw away leftover meals rather than trying to cool it and eat it later. Coolers are not efficient at cooling down hot food, and bacteria can multiply at a high rate in lukewarm food environments. Discard responsibly, being aware of wildlife, pests, and the natural environment.

When you get home, throw away any leftover food in the cooler, especially if the cooler no longer has solid ice to keep it cold enough.

Be aware of campground rules on how and where to dispose of wastewater from dishes, cooking, and self-care (like brushing teeth).

Adhere to all rules regarding fire. Some campgrounds allow fire in designated pits, some only allow camp stoves with a controlled flame that you can turn off, and some don't allow anything at all. If it is fire season or very dry, there may be burn bans in place. Plan for cooking in alternate ways, or eating foods that don't have to be cooked if this is the case.

Wash your hands before handling food and before eating. Dry hands with a designated towel separate from the dish towel.

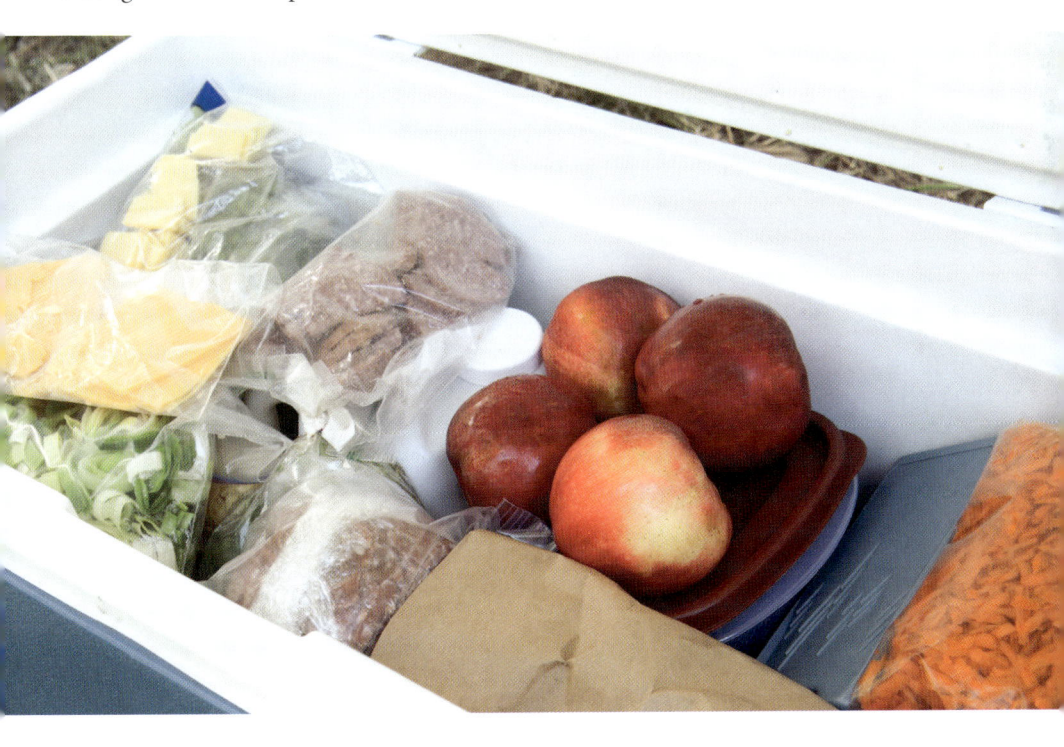

Research the water situation before leaving home. Does the campground provide potable water? Do you need to bring your own? Don't rely on streams or lakes for clean, safe water unless you plan on filtering all of the water you use. Only use potable water for any drinking, cooking, dishwashing, rinsing, brushing teeth, and other self-care.

SUGGESTED EQUIPMENT PACKING LIST

- Pan
- Pot
- Cooking utensils (spatula, spoon, etc.)
- Plates
- Bowls
- Eating utensils
- Mug
- Cup
- Camp stove
- Cooking fuel
- Matches or lighter
- Paper or cloth towel
- Soap
- Hand sanitizer
- Knife
- Cutting board
- Aluminum foil
- Food thermometer
- Trash bags
- Sanitizing wipes

SUGGESTED FOOD STAPLES

- Pasta
- Powdered mixes (pancake, milk, sauces, soups, etc.)
- Bread
- Peanut butter
- Jelly
- Oil or butter
- Canned meats and fish
- Jerky
- Trail mix
- Juice boxes
- Dried fruit
- Oatmeal

CAMPING MEAL IDEAS

The internet is full of camping meal ideas! Here are a few basic ones to get you started. These are classic go-tos because they are simple to prepare and only need a few ingredients.

- Spaghetti and meatballs
- Tacos, burritos, quesadillas, or taco salad
- Loaded baked potatoes

Foil dinners—meat cubes, corn, potato cubes, and seasonings packed in foil "pouch" and cooked over the coals

Chili

Chow mein

Pancakes, bacon, and eggs

French toast and diced potatoes or hash browns

Yogurt, granola, and fruit bowls

Oatmeal

Lasagna (cook in cast iron skillet over fire)

Sandwiches

Burgers or hot dogs

Breakfast hash

Pizza pockets

Kebabs/skewers

Breakfast sandwiches

Macaroni and cheese

Wraps

Teriyaki bowls

Ramen with meat, tofu, or boiled egg and choice of vegetables

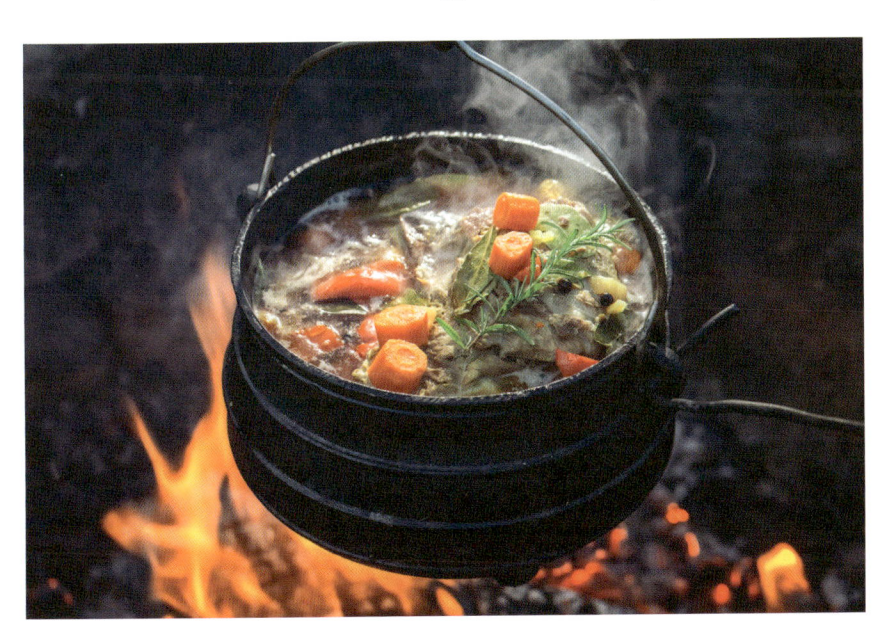

3-DAY SAMPLE CAMPING MENU

	Day 1	Day 2	Day 3
Breakfast	Breakfast burritos, melon	Pancakes, eggs, and melon	Yogurt with fruit and granola
Lunch	Build-your-own charcuterie with crackers, cheese, cured meat, olives, dried apricots, nuts, grapes	Turkey wraps, carrot sticks and hummus	Ramen with beef, soft-boiled egg, carrots, and spinach
Snack	Trail mix, apple	Bagel with peanut butter or cream cheese, grapes	Guacamole with chips and sliced cucumber and cherry tomatoes
Dinner	Spaghetti with marinara and ground beef, spinach salad	Chicken foil pouches roasted over campfire with diced potatoes, corn, carrots, and onion	Curry rice bowls with tofu, onion, spinach, carrots

DIY TRAIL MIX

Trail mix is always a classic! A tasty mix of sweet and salty, trail mix is a nice blend of carbs, fats, and proteins to fuel any outdoor adventure. Mix any ingredients according to your desired tastes and proportions.

- Pretzels
- Peanut butter–filled pretzel nuggets
- Yogurt-covered pretzels
- Goldfish crackers
- Sesame crackers
- Peanuts
- Almonds
- Cashews
- Pecans
- Hazelnuts
- Pistachios
- Macadamia nuts
- Sunflower seeds
- Pumpkin seeds
- Honey-roasted peanuts
- Yogurt-covered raisins
- Raisins
- Golden raisins
- Dried cranberries
- Dried blueberries
- Dried apricots
- Dried cherries
- Dried coconut flakes
- Dried strawberries
- Dried mangoes
- Dates
- Dried edamame
- Wasabi peas
- Banana chips
- Dried pineapple chunks
- Mini marshmallows
- M&Ms
- Whoppers (malted chocolate milk balls)
- Chocolate-covered almonds
- Gummy bears
- Gummy peach rings
- Chocolate chips
- White chocolate chips
- Yogurt chips
- Peanut butter chips
- Butterscotch chips
- Cheerios
- Chex
- Popcorn

Favorite combos:

The Classic: Peanuts, raisins, M&Ms

The Tropical: Macadamia nuts, coconut flakes, dried pineapple, dried apricot, white chocolate chips

The Spicy: Wasabi peas, sesame crackers, peanuts

The Fruit Salad: Dried cherries, dried apricots, dried mangoes, chocolate chips, almonds

The Inner Child: Cheerios, gummy bears, M&Ms, honey-roasted peanuts

S'MORES

While this is a book about nutrition for outdoor recreation, food isn't just for nutrition and fuel! It's also about connection, culture, tradition, and enjoyment. No camping trip is complete without s'mores around a campfire.

Take your s'mores up a notch with these ideas. Mix and match to make your own custom combinations.

Outer Layer	Marshmallow Layer	Chocolate Layer	Bonus Add-ins
Graham crackers	Marshmallow	Hershey's chocolate	Peanut butter
Chocolate graham crackers	Toasted coconut marshmallow	White chocolate	Cookie butter
Biscoff cookies	Fruity marshmallows	Caramel-filled chocolate squares	Brie
Nutter Butters	Gourmet marshmallows	Mint chocolate (Andes, Ghirardelli)	Thinly sliced apple, peach, or pineapple
Oreos (any flavor)	Marshmallow creme	Strawberry or raspberry chocolate squares	Mascarpone
Waffle cone cookie pieces	Peeps	Cookies n' cream Hershey's	Whipped cream
Chocolate chip cookies	Coconut macaroon		Nutella
Fudge shortbread cookies	Meringue		Caramel
Nilla wafer			Bacon
Chocolate mint cookies			Cookie dough
Rice Krispie treat			Ice cream
			Dulce de leche
			Lemon curd

Favorite combos:

Mint S'moreo: Mint Oreo + marshmallow

Berry Good: Waffle cone pieces + marshmallow + dark chocolate + smashed raspberry

Choco Coco Nut: Nutter Butter + coconut marshmallow + caramel chocolate square

Tropical Bliss: Nilla wafer + coconut marshmallow + chocolate + pineapple slice

THE WRAP-UP

Camping requires knowledge of safe food preparation and storage in order to make the trip a success. Special circumstances, such as high altitude or extreme heat or cold may alter your fueling and hydration needs. Bringing a variety of simple ingredients and basic cooking supplies streamlines meal prep.

REFERENCES

Arazi, H., A. Rashidlamir, M. Z. Abolhasani, and S. A. Hosanini. "Profiling and Predicting Performance of Indoor Rock Climbers." *Revista Brasileira de Cineantropometria e Desempenho Humano* 20, no. 1 (2018), 82–94.

Blunt-Gonzalez, G., L. Joubert, and A. Larson. "Differences in Perception of Body Weight and Fitness Components on Performance in Rock Climbers." Unpublished data, 2019. Personal communication, January 28, 2020.

Burke, L. M., and I. Mujika. "Nutrition for Recovery in Aquatic Sports." *International Journal of Sport Nutrition and Exercise Metabolism* 24, no. 4 (August 2014), 425–36. doi: 10.1123/ijsnem.2014-0022. Epub 2014 Jun 5. PMID: 24901517.

Chlíbková, D., B. Knechtle, T. Rosemann, I. Tomášková, V. Chadim, and M. Shortall. "Nutrition Habits in 24-Hour Mountain Bike Racers." *Springerplus* 3 (December 9, 2014), 715. doi: 10.1186/2193-1801-3-715. PMID: 25674455; PMCID: PMC4320206.

Costa, R. J. S., B. Knechtle, M. Tarnopolsky, and M. D. Hoffman. "Nutrition for Ultramarathon Running: Trail, Track, and Road." *International Journal of Sport Nutrition and Exercise Metabolism* 29, no. 2 (March 1, 2019), 130–40. doi: 10.1123/ijsnem.2018-0255. Epub 2019 Apr 3. PMID: 30943823.

Giles, D., K. Barnes, N. Taylor, C. Chidley, J. Chidley, J. Mitchell, O. Torr, E. Gibson-Smith, and V. España-Romero. "Anthropometry and Performance Characteristics of Recreational Advanced to Elite Female Rock Climbers." *Journal of Sports Sciences* 39, no. 1 (January 2, 2021), 48–56.

Grønhaug, G. "Lean and Mean? Associations of Level of Performance, Chronic Injuries and BMI in Sport Climbing." *BMJ Open Sport & Exercise Medicine* 5, no. 1 (2019), e000437.

Herrmann, S. D., E. A. Willis, B. E. Ainsworth, T. V. Barreira, M. Hastert, C. L. Kracht, J. M. Schuna Jr., Z. Cai, M. Quan, C. Tudor-Locke, M. C. Whitt-Glover, and D. R. Jacobs Jr. "2024 Adult Compendium of Physical

Activities: A Third Update of the Energy Costs of Human Activities." *Journal of Sport and Health Science* 13, no. 1 (January 2024), 6–12. doi: 10.1016/j.jshs.2023.10.010. PMID: 38242596; PMCID: PMC10818145.

Impellizzeri, F. M., and S. M. Marcora. "The Physiology of Mountain Biking." *Sports Medicine* 37, no. 1 (2007), 59–71. doi: 10.2165/00007256-200737010-00005. PMID: 17190536.

Jeukendrup, A. E., R. L. Jentjens, and L. Moseley. "Nutritional Considerations in Triathlon." *Sports Medicine* 35, no. 2 (2005), 163–81. doi: 10.2165/00007256-200535020-00005. PMID: 15707379.

Jiménez-Casquet, M. J., J. Conde-Pipó, I. Valenzuela-Barranco, R. Rienda-Contreras, F. Olea-Serrano, C. Bouzas, J. A. Tur, and M. Mariscal-Arcas. "Nutrition Status of Female Winter Sports Athletes." *Nutrients* 15, no. 20 (October 22, 2023), 4472. doi: 10.3390/nu15204472. PMID: 37892548; PMCID: PMC10609974.

Karpęcka-Gałka, E., P. Mazur-Kurach, Z. Szyguła, and B. Frączek. "Diet, Supplementation and Nutritional Habits of Climbers in High Mountain Conditions." *Nutrients* 15, no. 19 (September 29, 2023), 4219. doi: 10.3390/nu15194219. PMID: 37836503; PMCID: PMC10574574.

Kim, J., and E. K. Kim. "Nutritional Strategies to Optimize Performance and Recovery in Rowing Athletes." *Nutrients* 12, no. 6 (June 5, 2020), 1685. doi: 10.3390/nu12061685. PMID: 32516908; PMCID: PMC7352678.

Laffaye, G., J. M. Collin, and G. Levernier. "Determinant Factors in Climbing Ability; Influence of Strength, Anthropometry, and Neuromuscular Fatigue." *Scandinavian Journal of Medicine and Science in Sports* 26, no. 10 (2015), 1151–59.

Laval, I. L., and S. Sitko. "Performance Factors in Sport Climbing and Bouldering: Systematic Review." *Journal of Sports Training* 33, no. 3 (2019).

Looney, D. P., E. M. Lavoie, S. V. Vangala, L. D. Holden, P. S. Figueiredo, K. E. Friedl, P. N. Frykman, J. W. Hancock, S. J. Montain, J. L. Pryor, W. R. Santee, and A. W. Potter. "Modeling the Metabolic Costs of Heavy Military Backpacking." *Medicine and Science in Sports and Exercise* 54, no. 4 (April 1, 2022), 646–54. doi: 10.1249/MSS.0000000000002833. PMID: 34856578; PMCID: PMC8919998.

Mermier, C. M., J. M. Janot, D. L. Parker, and J. G. Swan. "Physiological and Anthropometric Determinants of Sport Climbing Performance." *British Journal of Sports Medicine* 34 (2000), 359–66.

Meyer, N. L., M. M. Manore, and C. Helle. "Nutrition for Winter Sports." *Journal of Sports Sciences* 29, suppl. 1 (2011), S127–36. doi: 10.1080/02640414.2011.574721. Epub 2011 Jun 21. PMID: 22150424.

Michael, M. *Nutrition for Climbers: Fuel for the Send*. Boulder, CO: Fixed Pin Publishing, LLC, 2020.

Michael, M. K., L. Joubert, and O. C. Witard. "Assessment of Dietary Intake and Eating Attitudes in Recreational and Competitive Adolescent Rock Climbers: A Pilot Study." *Frontiers in Nutrition* 6 (2019), 64.

Michael, M. K., O. C. Witard, L. Joubert, and R. Taiar. "Physiological Demands and Nutritional Considerations for Olympic-Style Competitive Rock Climbing." *Cogent Medicine* 6. no. 1 (2019). doi: https://doi.org/10.1080/2331205X.2019.1667199.

Ozimek, M., R. Rokowski, P. Draga, V. Ljakh, T. Ambroźy, M. Krawczyk, T. Ręgwelski, A. Stanula, K. Görner, A. Jurczak, and D. Mucha. "The Role of Physique, Strength, and Endurance in the Achievements of Elite Climbers." *PLoS One* 12, no. 8 (2017), e0182026.

Ranchordas, M. K. "Nutrition for Adventure Racing," *Sports Medicine* 42, no. 11 (November 1, 2012), 915–27. doi: 10.1007/BF03262303. PMID: 23006142.

Saenz, C., A. Jordan, L. Loriz, K. Schill, M. Colletto, and J. Rodriguez. "Low Energy Intake Leads to Body Composition and Performance Decrements in a Highly-Trained, Female Athlete: The WANDER (Woman's Activity and Nutrition during an Extensive Hiking Route) Case Study." *Journal of the American Nutrition Association* 43, no. 3 (March-April 2024), 296–303. doi: 10.1080/27697061.2023.2282614. Epub 2023 Nov 29. PMID: 38019616.

Saul, D., G. Steinmetz, W. Lehmann, and A. F. Schilling. "Determinants for Success in Climbing: A Systematic Review." *Journal of Exercise Science & Fitness* 17, no. 3 (September 1, 2019), 91–100. https://doi.org/10.1016/j.jesf.2019.04.002.

Shaw, G., K. T. Boyd, L. M. Burke, and A. Koivisto. "Nutrition for Swimming." *International Journal of Sport Nutrition and Exercise Metabolism* 24, no. 4 (August 2014), 360–72. doi: 10.1123/ijsnem.2014-0015. Epub 2014 Jun 5. PMID: 24903758.

Shaw, G., A. Koivisto, D. Gerrard, and L. M. Burke. "Nutrition Considerations for Open-Water Swimming." *International Journal of Sport Nutrition and*

Exercise Metabolism 24, no. 4 (August 2014), 373–81. doi: 10.1123/ijsnem.2014-0018. Epub 2014 Mar 25. PMID: 24667305.

Stellingwerff, T., D. B. Pyne, and L. M. Burke. "Nutrition Considerations in Special Environments for Aquatic Sports." *International Journal of Sport Nutrition and Exercise Metabolism* 24, no. 4 (August 2014), 470–79. doi: 10.1123/ijsnem.2014-0014. Epub 2014 Jun 17. PMID: 24937361.

Tiller, N. B., J. D. Roberts, L. Beasley, S. Chapman, J. M. Pinto, L. Smith, M. Wiffin, M. Russell, S. A. Sparks, L. Duckworth, J. O'Hara, L. Sutton, J. Antonio, D. S. Willoughby, M. D. Tarpey, A. E. Smith-Ryan, M. J. Ormsbee, T. A. Astorino, R. B. Kreider, G. R. McGinnis, J. R. Stout, J. W. Smith, S. M. Arent, B. I. Campbell, and L. Bannock. "International Society of Sports Nutrition Position Stand: Nutritional Considerations for Single-Stage Ultra-Marathon Training and Racing. *Journal of the International Society of Sports Nutrition* 16, no. 1 (November 7, 2019), 50. doi: 10.1186/s12970-019-0312-9. PMID: 31699159; PMCID: PMC6839090.

6
DISORDERED EATING AND RELATIVE ENERGY DEFICIENCY IN SPORT (REDs)

This may seem like a strange topic to include in a book on nutrition for outdoor recreation, but I would be amiss if I did not include a chapter on disordered eating and relative energy deficiency in sport (REDs). These two conditions are common in athletic populations. Not only elite athletes can be affected. Anyone from the 9-year-old youth snowboarder to the 50-year-old ultrarunner could struggle with these conditions.

It is vitally important to be educated about disordered eating and REDs. Both can result in mild decreased health and performance outcomes, to—in the most severe cases—permanent infertility, osteoporosis, and even death.

The information in this chapter will support our overarching goals for the book:

- Eat enough to support basic body processes.
- Eat enough to support training and movement (before, during, and after activity).
- Eat a healthful diet made of mostly whole grains, fruits/vegetables, nuts/seeds, dairy products, and lean protein.
- Refuel and rehydrate after workouts to promote recovery.
- Maintain a good relationship with food, body, and sport.

This last goal especially relates to this chapter. You will learn:

- What are eating disorders vs. disordered eating?
- Types, signs, and symptoms of eating disorders
- All about relative energy deficiency in sport (REDs)
- Health and performance outcomes of these conditions
- Signs/symptoms of these conditions
- Relation of body weight to sports performance
- How to foster a good relationship with food, body, and sport

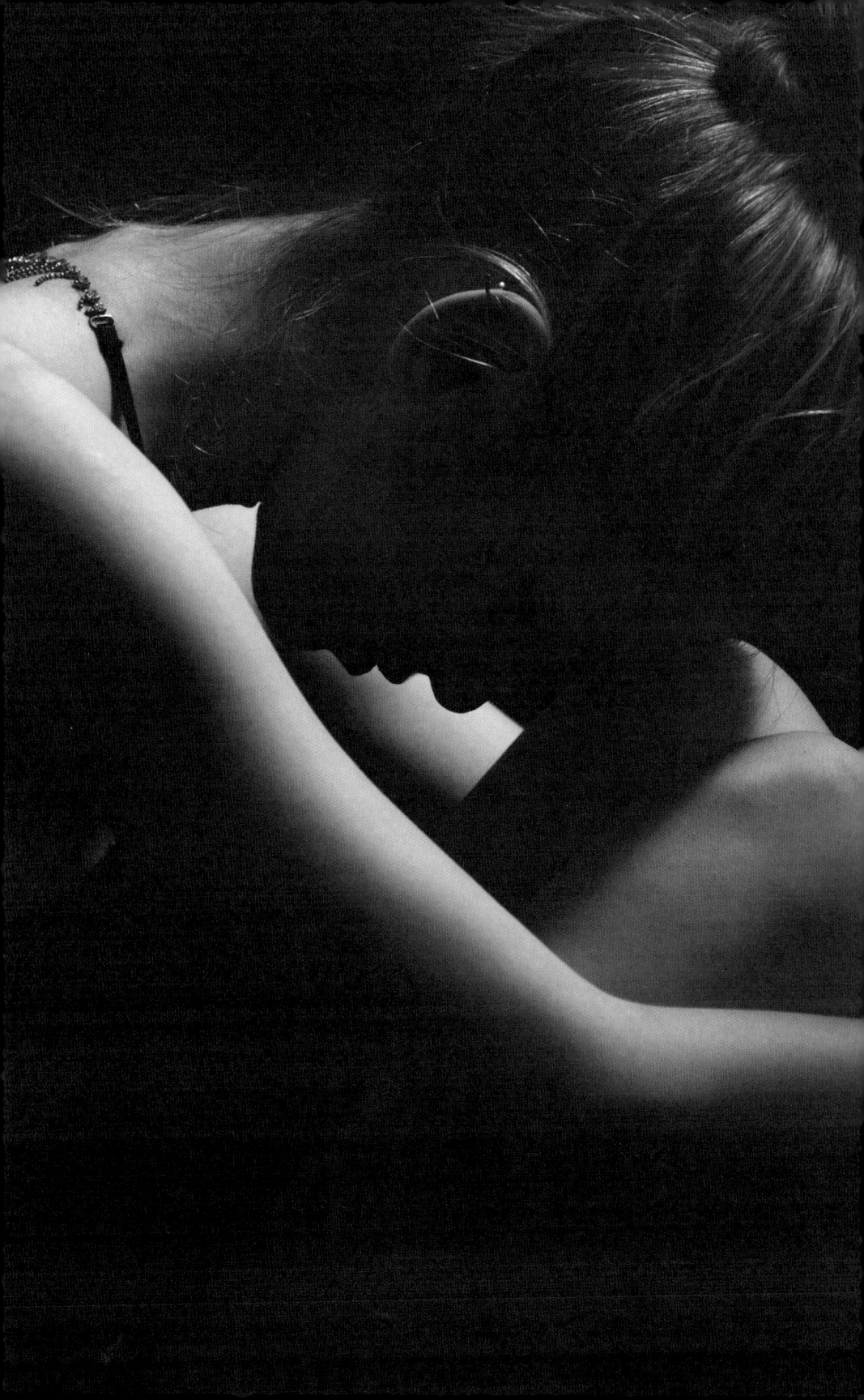

Amelia Boone, an accomplished obstacle racer and endurance athlete, writes about her struggles with anorexia nervosa in *Outside* magazine. She describes years of missing her period, being diagnosed with osteopenia (low bone density) at age 16, multiple stress fractures—all the while winning races and appearing to be in peak physical condition. The message is clear: You don't know who is struggling, and you can't judge whether someone has an eating disorder based on looks or performance.

Unfortunately, stories like hers are all too common in the sports world. If you find yourself relating to this section, seek professional help from an informed and well-trained sports nutrition professional. Even if you think it may be no big deal, or you aren't sick enough to justify medical care, the conditions described here are serious and you deserve treatment.

EATING DISORDER VS. DISORDERED EATING

While these two phrases seem similar, it is important to understand the distinction. An *eating disorder* is a clinical diagnosis with specific criteria based on the *Diagnostic and Statistical Manual of Mental Disorders, 5th Edition* (DSM-5). *Disordered eating* refers to disordered eating patterns that don't necessarily fit certain diagnostic measures. Since eating patterns fall on a spectrum, some may be considered disordered, while others fit a formal diagnosis.

Both are harmful to mental and physical health. Both can be serious and even fatal. For the purposes of this section, I will be using the phrase *disordered eating* to refer to any disrupted eating patterns, including those that are a diagnosable illness.

Disordered eating is primarily a mental illness, but has physical effects depending on the type, severity, and duration of the illness. Any type of disordered eating needs correct treatment in order to recover fully. This usually includes a team of a doctor, a dietitian, and a therapist.

It is vital to seek treatment early and stay with the treatment until the person is in recovery.

EATING DISORDERS

Anorexia nervosa

This is probably the most commonly known eating disorder. People with anorexia restrict their food intake in an effort to be thinner. They often have body dysmorphia (which is a distorted view of their own body). They may also compulsively exercise and increase movement in order to lose weight. Anorexia nervosa has the second-highest mortality rate after opioid use. Health complications can be severe, permanent, and life-threatening.

Some signs and symptoms of anorexia include:

- Rapid and/or extreme weight loss
- Behavioral changes
- Mood disturbances
- Attempt to purge calories by laxatives and/or excessive exercise
- Hair loss or thinning
- Sensitivity to cold
- Fatigue
- Lost or irregular periods
- Dizziness, especially when going from sitting to standing
- Strange eating habits or food rituals, such as separating all foods on the plate, or cutting up food into tiny pieces
- Intense fear of becoming fat
- Obsession with eating, counting calories, or any kind of diet

Health complications from anorexia can include:

- Irregular heart rhythms and cardiac arrest
- Heart, kidney, or liver failure
- Loss of bone density, osteoporosis, and increased risk of fracture
- Gastrointestinal issues, such as bloating, constipation, malabsorption, and food intolerances
- Loss of period or irregular periods
- Infertility
- Anemia

Bulimia Nervosa

This is characterized by a cycle of food restriction, bingeing, and purging. Use of vomiting, laxatives, sweat suits, saunas, or excessive exercise are all forms of purging. The main goal of purging is weight loss and/or getting rid of perceived excess calories to prevent weight gain. Some people have body dysmorphia as well.

Bulimia is also a serious disease that can cause profound health complications and death.

Some signs and symptoms of bulimia are:

- Consuming large amounts of food, usually rapidly and in secret with feeling of loss of control (this is a binge)
- Guilt and shame associated with the binge episode
- Slow heart rate
- Dizziness and/or low blood pressure, especially when going from sitting to standing
- Vomiting, spitting food out, laxative, and diuretic use
- Swelling in the cheeks or jaw (from vomiting)
- Scars on the backs of the hands (from vomiting)
- Frequent use of the bathroom after meals (to go vomit)
- Fear of gaining weight
- Change in social routines or withdrawal from friends and family
- Worsening performance at school, sports, work, or other activities

Health complications from bulimia can include:

- Irregular heartbeat
- Heart failure
- Electrolyte imbalances
- Dehydration
- Edema (swelling in ankles from water retention)
- Ulcers
- Pancreatitis
- Tooth decay and esophageal damage from vomiting
- Digestive problems
- Fatigue

Binge Eating Disorder (BED)

This disorder is distinct from bulimia in that it does not have a purging component. Some people experience night eating syndrome, which is overeating during the night or waking to eat large quantities of food. Both bulimia and night eating syndrome can be treated with medication, nutrition therapy, mental health therapy, and the oversight of a doctor.

Bingeing is hard to specifically define, but it is different than simply overeating when you are hungry, or feeling like you ate a lot one day due to a holiday, vacation, or simply being extra hungry. A binge often feels compulsive and uncontrollable. Some people report feeling like they are dissociated during the binge, and don't have any sense of how much or what they are eating. When they "come out of it" they realize there are lots of dishes and food wrappers around. Binges are more than just a large meal. They are a large volume of food that most people could not eat in one sitting. After the binge, the digestive system is usually very painful or uncomfortable with bloating, upset stomach, heartburn, and irregular bowel movements.

Here are some signs and symptoms of BED:

- Eating very rapidly
- Eating until feeling very full, uncomfortably so
- Eating large amounts of food even when not hungry
- Eating alone to hide the amount of food eaten
- Feelings of guilt, embarrassment, shame, or disgust with oneself after bingeing

Here are some health consequences that can occur with BED:

- High cholesterol
- High blood pressure
- Increased risk for heart disease and Type 2 diabetes
- Gastrointestinal problems, such as constipation, diarrhea, and acid reflux

Avoidant Restrictive Food Intake Disorder (ARFID)

This eating disorder has a restrictive component, but it is not due to a drive for thinness or a desire to manipulate body weight, composition, shape, or size. Instead, it is often labeled as "picky eating" but goes beyond that, to the point that nutrient deficiencies and malnourishment can result.

The "picky eating" is usually due to sensitive taste or texture issues, where many foods are undesirable to the person. It can also be due to a past food trauma, such as choking on many foods as a toddler and then avoiding those foods as a teen or adult, even though it is now safe to eat them.

People with ARFID usually have very narrow foods they are able to eat, such as only pasta, bread, and chicken nuggets. They have extreme difficulty trying new foods, and sometimes have negative intense reactions to new foods. This type of eating disorder needs a treatment team of a doctor, dietitian, and therapist that are well trained in exposure therapy and other methods to help the person feel safe and expand their food options.

Some signs and symptoms of ARFID include:

- Extreme pickiness
- Food refusal
- Choking, gagging, or poor experience with food
- Fear of choking, gagging, or an allergic reaction
- Food avoidance due to sensory issues such as taste, texture, or appearance
- Lack of appetite
- Disinterest in eating
- Failure to grow in children
- Weight loss

Some health consequences that can occur with ARFID are:

- Heart issues
- Failure to grow in children
- Decreased training adaptations
- Weight loss
- Kidney and liver failure
- Anemia
- Electrolyte imbalances
- Digestive issues
- Fatigue, fainting, lightheadedness
- Hair loss
- Difficulty concentrating

Other Specified Feeding and Eating Disorders (OSFED)

This is a category of eating disorders that do not fit the other diagnoses. It also includes compulsive exercise and body dysmorphic disorder. Many of these signs and symptoms share commonality with other eating disorders.

Here are some signs and symptoms of OSFED:

- Dieting by restricting calories or whole food groups
- Excessive exercise
- Purging with laxatives, diuretics, vomiting, or excessive exercise
- Distorted body image

- Strange food behaviors such as cutting food into tiny pieces or having many food rules
- Obsession with eating "clean," "pure," or "perfect"
- Shame, anxiety, and guilt associated with eating
- Hiding behaviors or feeling a loss of control over behaviors, such as eating to be overly full, hiding food, or bingeing at night when no one can witness the binge

Here are some health consequences that can occur with OSFED:

- Unintended extreme weight loss or gain
- High or low blood pressure
- High or low blood sugar (especially in those with diabetes)
- Missing nutrients in one's diet
- Anemia

Orthorexia

This is not an official diagnosis, but it is worth mentioning here because the health consequences and emotional impact can be just as real and severe as other "official" eating disorders. It is viewed as the pursuit of eating "clean," "healthy," or "perfect" to the extent that it interferes with someone's day-to-day life. It is a strong obsession with only eating foods deemed healthy by self-imposed rules.

People with orthorexia often spend large amounts of time procuring, cooking, and eating the food. They may have a very large grocery bill because they only buy foods according to their own rules, such as avoiding certain ingredients, only eating organic, or avoiding certain food groups.

They often struggle to find "acceptable" foods in social situations, restaurants, while traveling, or around holiday celebrations. They have rigid rules and would rather not eat than eat food that does not comply with the rules. If they break a rule, they often feel guilt, shame, or anxiety.

Orthorexia is sometimes a way to cope with anxiety, it is sometimes motivated by health, or can also be an ill-informed person that believes "healthy food" fits into their narrow rules.

Dr. Steve Bratman coined the term *orthorexia* and has the following quiz available to self-assess:

1. I spend so much of my life thinking about, choosing, and preparing healthy food that it interferes with other dimensions of my life, such as love, creativity, family, friendship, work, and school.

2. When I eat any food I regard to be unhealthy, I feel anxious, guilty, impure, unclean, and/or defiled; even to be near such foods disturbs me, and I feel judgmental of others who eat such foods.
3. My personal sense of peace, happiness, joy, safety, and self-esteem is excessively dependent on the purity and righteousness of what I eat.
4. Sometimes I would like to relax my self-imposed "good food" rules for a special occasion, such as a wedding or a meal with family and friends, but I find that I cannot. (Note: if you have a medical condition in which it is unsafe for you to make *any* exception to your diet, then this item does not apply.)
5. Over time, I have steadily eliminated more foods and expanded my list of food rules in an attempt to maintain or enhance health benefits; sometimes, I may take an existing food theory and add to it with beliefs of my own.
6. Following my theory of healthy eating has caused me to lose more weight than most people would say is good for me or has caused other signs of malnutrition such as hair loss, loss of menstruation, or skin problems.

A "yes" answer to any of these questions means you may have or be developing orthorexia.

The following signs and symptoms of orthorexia are from the National Eating Disorder Association website:

- Compulsive checking of ingredient lists and nutritional labels
- An increase in concern about the health of ingredients
- Cutting out an increasing number of food groups (all sugar, all carbs, all dairy, all meat, all animal products)
- An inability to eat anything but a narrow group of foods that are deemed "healthy" or "pure"
- Unusual interest in the health of what others are eating
- A feeling of superiority around their nutrition and intolerance of other people's food behaviors and beliefs
- High levels of perfectionism
- Spending hours per day thinking about what food might be served at upcoming events

- Showing high levels of distress when "safe" or "healthy" foods aren't available
- Obsessive following of food and "healthy lifestyle" blogs on social media
- Body image concerns may or may not be present
- Psychosocial impairments in different areas of life

RELATIVE ENERGY DEFICIENCY IN SPORT (REDs)

Relative energy deficiency in sport (REDs) is a condition where there is a mismatch between energy intake and energy expenditure. Simply put, it means your exercise output is higher than your calorie intake. This energy deficit can lead to several health complications over time.

If your body is in a state of low energy availability, this means it is not getting enough food to fuel all the normal body processes, plus exercise and activities of daily living. This is a simplistic view, but a helpful starting point to understanding REDs.

An easy analogy is to think of it like a budget and paying bills. Your body's basal metabolism demands some energy. Things like breathing, the heart beating, normal cell turnover (intestines, bones, etc.), immune system function, and reproductive function (menstruation, sex hormone production, etc.) all take energy. This energy comes from calories you eat in your food. These mandatory "bills" need to be paid.

Now layer in everything else you do in a day. Thinking, household chores, meeting with coworkers, walking, sitting—anything you do beyond lying down requires more energy in addition to the energy you already need for basal metabolism. More "bills" that must be paid.

Then on top of this, add your purposeful exercise. Lifting at the gym, hiking, skiing, walking, swimming—anything—demands even more energy. These are optional "bills" that become mandatory if you make your body do these activities even when you're in an energy deficit.

If you don't eat enough to support all that you're asking your body to do, it must tighten its "budget." Since you are still hiking, working, and cleaning the house, your body must supply energy to make these tasks happen. Where can it cut some corners? What is left in the budget?

Your body has no choice but to make some cutbacks. Unfortunately, these cutbacks can lead to health problems. The mandatory "bills" like basal metabolism, hormone production, and immune maintenance are now compromised. You ran out of money paying the "hiking" bill, and now you can't pay the "heartbeat" bill.

Health Consequences of REDs	Signs of REDs
Decreased immunity	Frequent illness (colds, flu, etc.)
Decreased hormones	Low thyroid, low testosterone, low estrogen, missing or irregular periods, infertility
Decreased bone density	Low bone density when tested, stress fractures, slow healing of bone injury
Mental health issues	Depression, anxiety, mood swings, feeling "flat," lost motivation in sport or life, difficulty concentrating
Gastrointestinal complications	Constipation, diarrhea, bloating, runner's trots, low appetite, early satiety
Decreased muscle strength	Loss or plateau in training, decreased power
Weakened soft tissues	Tendon or ligament injuries, slower healing time
Disrupted sleep	Having trouble falling asleep or staying asleep
Impaired cardiovascular function	Resting heart rate below 40 bpm, abnormal EKG, feeling lightheaded or heart rate too high when going from sitting to standing
Impaired growth in children and adolescents	Falling off growth curve, not hitting expected full adult height
Fatigue, increased risk of cardiac disease	Anemia, low thyroid, low leptin, high cholesterol, and abnormal blood lab values

Potential performance outcomes of REDs:

- Decreased power
- Decreased endurance
- Decreased strength
- Poor recovery
- Decreased or arrested training response
- Decreased coordination
- Decreased concentration
- Decreased motivation

As you can see from this information, REDs can have serious health and performance consequences. The main message is this: *Eat enough food!* How do you know what "enough" is? Go to Chapter 1 for more information or visit with a sports dietitian to nail down a personalized nutrition plan.

There is growing evidence that REDs could be the result of not just low energy availability, but low *carbohydrate* availability. The body certainly needs enough energy (from your food and fluid intake) in order to function properly and do all the sports you ask it to do. But it also needs carbohydrate! Athletes that restrict carbohydrate or accidentally under-eat their carbohydrate are at risk for these REDs symptoms as well.

Even more fascinating, within-day low energy availability can also disrupt your normal body processes. Going too long without eating, skipping meals, intermittent fasting, or restricting your intake can all lead to low energy availability, even if your overall calorie intake is adequate.

Even those people without a diagnosable case of REDs can still have periods of low energy availability (or low carbohydrate availability) where symptoms like poor sleep, poor recovery, niggling pains, and small injuries start to appear.

REDs symptoms are usually multi-factorial. Stressors on the body, such as too little food, increased training, life stress, emotional issues, a difficult job or school load, illness, or injury can all contribute to REDs symptoms. They may be alleviated by adequate food or a decreased training load, but all other factors need to be considered.

For example, if you are experiencing poor sports performance, a tendon injury, a missing period, or anything else mentioned above, you may want to consider:

- Are you eating enough to match the training load?
- Are you eating enough carbs?
- Are you getting enough sleep?
- Do you have extra stress in your life, and is it possible to reduce it?
- Have you had a recent illness you're not yet fully recovered from?

REDs should not be dismissed. It can leave profound and permanent damage, and even death in the most extreme cases. Even in more mild cases, REDs should be addressed. This will help you feel and perform much better, as well as protect your health in both the short and long term.

> **FEMALE ATHLETE TRIAD**
>
> The female athlete triad concept was developed decades ago when clinicians started noticing a similar pattern in some female athletes: osteoporosis, disordered eating, and amenorrhea (missing period).
>
> As more research was done, they also observed that female athletes didn't always have the extreme cases of both amenorrhea, osteoporosis, and disordered eating, but some were experiencing negative health effects with milder symptoms, such as osteopenia and irregular periods. They still used the term *female athlete triad* to describe this syndrome, but now it was recognized that it existed on a spectrum.
>
> It wasn't until 2014 that the International Olympic Committee published a landmark paper describing REDs. It was clear at this point that the female athlete triad was more than just a "triad"—multiple negative health outcomes were stemming from under-eating. And it wasn't just females who were affected. People of all genders can suffer from REDs.
>
> In addition, one of the main components of the triad—disordered eating—was really just the *cause* of the osteoporosis and amenorrhea. This is because disordered eating resulted in low energy availability. The mismatch between energy intake and energy expenditure is the underlying cause of female athlete triad and REDs.
>
> You may still see the term *female athlete triad* used today by some people, but this is an outdated term that no longer describes the condition accurately. The root cause of the symptoms is from not eating enough food: Whether that is caused by disordered eating or by inadvertently not eating enough, the physical impact is still the same.

The treatment for this complex syndrome is actually very simple, cost effective, and accessible: Eat more food and/or reduce exercise, and reduce total body stress. Although the treatment is simple, implementing the treatment takes specialized support and is best done with a professional. Seek out a doctor and dietitian trained in REDs for the best outcomes.

DISORDERED EATING AND REDs

You may be wondering: Can someone get REDs from disordered eating? Is REDs only caused by disordered eating?

REDs is caused by not eating enough to match energy expenditure. Whether this occurs due to disordered eating, purposeful dieting, or inadvertent under-eating, or a high stress load, the health outcomes can be the same.

Not all people with REDs have disordered eating, and not all disordered eating may lead to REDs. However, someone with disordered eating—especially a restrictive type—could have REDs as a result.

OVERTRAINING AND REDs

Overtraining syndrome closely matches many signs and symptoms of REDs. So, if someone is experiencing these symptoms, is it overtraining, or is it REDs? There is evidence in the scientific literature that overtraining may be prevented in some cases by eating enough. Matching energy and carbohydrate intake to the training load is vital to see good training adaptations.

In many studies, athletes tend to increase their training load without increasing their food intake to match the higher training load. Preventing REDs and overtraining takes diligence and awareness. If you are increasing training duration, frequency, or intensity, you need to also eat more to compensate for that increased energy expenditure.

Diagnosing overtraining and REDs is complex. Seek medical expertise if you suspect either syndrome.

RELATIONSHIP OF BODY WEIGHT TO SPORTS PERFORMANCE

Many sports involve some level of fighting gravity. From ski jumping to rock climbing, cycling to running, and hiking up mountains with a pack—we all have experienced that feeling that you wish your body, your backpack, or your equipment felt lighter.

An optimized strength-to-weight ratio is often seen as the holy grail of sports performance. However, this isn't always the case, even in sports where fighting gravity is the norm.

Physics demands certain conditions to create peak performance. Less friction on a road bike tire and less weight in your pack on a thru-hike means you may go faster with more efficiency. But this doesn't necessarily mean you need to lose weight or body fat in order to achieve peak performance.

Having an appropriate body weight and amount of body fat can help your body function optimally. Weight loss for the sake of optimizing your sport's physics may be detrimental. Weight and body composition are only one tiny piece of the performance puzzle. To manipulate both is fraught with barriers and risks, such as:

- Underperformance due to under-fueling
- Loss of lean muscle mass
- Decreased hormone function

- Increased risk of disordered eating
- Fatigue
- Loss of concentration and focus
- Increased risk of illness and injury

If you are already in an appropriate weight range, focusing on other variables for sports performance will likely benefit you more than attempting weight loss. Other variables could include:

- Increasing strength
- Increasing flexibility
- Increasing endurance
- Enhancing sport-specific skills
- Dialing in your nutrition and hydration strategy
- Adapting the appropriate training plan
- Periodizing training and rest/recovery
- Ensuring adequate sleep
- Selectively choosing evidence-based supplements

Besides aspects like strength, flexibility, endurance, and skill, many other factors impact sports performance:

- Weather (cold, heat, humidity)
- Altitude
- Years of experience in the sport
- Hours of training per week in the sport
- Mindset/motivation
- Nutrition/hydration
- Genetics
- Equipment/gear
- Sleep quality and duration
- Mental toughness
- Recovery/rest
- Medical conditions
- Some medications
- Menstrual status
- Reaction time

It's important to take all these into consideration, rather than a knee-jerk reaction ("If I lost weight, I bet I'd be better"). And remember, weight is just one side of the "strength-to-weight ratio" concept. If you're involved in a sport that demands a high strength-to-weight ratio, rather than focusing on weight loss, what if you focused on strength? How would that change your performance? This is usually a much better approach with less risk than weight loss.

HOW TO FOSTER A GOOD RELATIONSHIP WITH FOOD/BODY/EXERCISE

A good relationship with your body can serve as a solid foundation for choices you make around food and exercise. Honoring your body and making decisions from a place of self-care are key concepts to having a good relationship with food, your own body, and your exercise patterns. A poor relationship with food, body, or exercise can lead to choices that may be detrimental to mental and physical health.

This may be an abstract concept, so let's use real-life examples to illustrate what this means.

WHICH SIDE STANDS OUT TO YOU?

Take a look at both sides of this chart. See which side resonates with you the most. Are there any habits you could improve?

Healthy Relationship with Food	Unhealthy Relationship with Food
Food as fuel, culture, celebration. Seeking athletic excellence through good nutrition.	Anxious about how much, when, and what to eat.
Food can be for enjoyment and pleasure.	Use food to cope with emotions.
Flexibility and variety in food choices.	Rigidity and restriction in food choices.
Using internal cues to guide food intake: tuning into hunger and fullness.	Using external cues to guide food intake: time of day, portion size, diet rules, etc.
Satisfaction with food choices and amount eaten.	Guilt, shame, or regret with food choices.

Dr. Kate Bennett, a sports psychologist at Athlete Insight, created a graphic that represents this same concept with exercise. The table above is based on Dr. Bennett's work and was originally published in *Nutrition for Climbers* (Fixed Pin Publishing). Used with permission.

Can you spot the difference between a good relationship and a poor relationship? A good relationship with food, body, and exercise allows for self-care, honoring your body's needs, and allowing flexibility with food intake and exercise plans. It is free of judgment, guilt, anxiety, and shame. It is wise and trusts body cues to guide decisions.

There is curiosity around actions. For example, if someone finds themselves eating cookies, ice cream, and chips after dinner, there is no judgment. There is curiosity—why am I doing this behavior? Overeating at night could be because:

- I under-fed myself today by only having coffee for breakfast. My body must be asking for more food.
- My last diet forbade cookies, and now that I am done with my diet I can't get enough of them. The restriction has made me crave them more, and also see them as a "bad" food.
- My parents didn't allow sweets in my house as a child. Now I want them all the time.
- I had a bad day and fought with a loved one. It feels good to soothe emotions with food.

These are just a few examples of how having a good relationship with food and body can help you learn to adopt more healthful behaviors in a non-judgmental way.

If you find yourself struggling with your food/body/sport relationships, seeking professional help can be really useful. Try to find a therapist, dietitian, and/or doctor that is informed in disordered eating recovery. Even if you don't have an eating disorder, professionals with this type of background are specially trained to help support you in healing your own relationship with food.

If you or someone you care about may have disordered eating, you can reach out to organizations such as the National Eating Disorders Association (nationaleatingdisorders.org), the National Association of Anorexia Nervosa and Associated Disorders (anad.org), or the Academy for Eating Disorders (aedweb.org). If you suspect something, say something. Eating disorders can be life-threatening and should not go without treatment.

Scenario	Poor Relationship	Good Relationship
A runner is feeling sick, but their training plan has a tempo run today and the race is 4 weeks away.	Do the run. Feel terrible.	Skip the run. Allow the body time to rest and recover. Recognize that running while sick will not lead to meaningful training gains, and skipping one run will not matter over the course of a training block.
A hiker has significant knee pain, but has a hike planned and also is in a weight loss phase.	Take the pain medicine. Hike because it can burn a lot of calories and the hiker is worried about body fat.	Skip the hike or seek physical therapy to better assess knee pain and get a recovery plan in place. Realize that exercise and food should not be a transactional relationship.
Meal prep on weekends to have lunches for work on the weekdays.	Meal prep because you need to stick to rigid diet rules that the meals comply with.	Meal prep because you notice that it helps to have healthful, nourishing foods ready to eat and it helps you feel energized for the workday.
Track calories and macros in an app.	Track because of anxiety and need to control food intake, body weight, or body composition. Feel shame or guilt when you don't track, or when you don't hit your goals.	Track to feel empowered to understand how to feed your body an appropriate amount of calories, protein, and carbohydrate, because when you are well fueled you feel and perform better. Don't track because you want to use body cues such as hunger, fullness, and satisfaction to help guide your food intake.

THE WRAP-UP

Disordered eating, eating disorders, and relative energy deficiency in sport are serious conditions that require professional support. Being aware of the signs and symptoms of each can help keep you safe and performing your best. Having a good relationship with food, body image, and exercise can help you make appropriate choices regarding diet and training.

REFERENCES

Boone, A. "Amelia Boone Opens Up About Her Eating Disorder." *Outside*, July 12, 2019. https://www.outsideonline.com/2399654/amelia-boone-eating-disorder.

Dvořáková, K., A. C. Paludo, A. Wagner, D. Puda, M. Gimunová, and M. Kumstát. "A Literature Review of Biomarkers Used for Diagnosis of Relative Energy Deficiency in Sport." *Frontiers in Sports and Active Living* 6 (July 12, 2024), 1375740. doi: 10.3389/fspor.2024.1375740. PMID: 39070233; PMCID: PMC11273787. https://www.nationaleatingdisorders.org/orthorexia/.

la Torre, M .E., A. Monda, A. Messina, M. I. de Stefano, V. Monda, F. Moscatelli, F. Tafuri, E. Saraiello, F. Latino, M. Monda, G. Messina, R. Polito, and D. Tafuri. "The Potential Role of Nutrition in Overtraining Syndrome: A Narrative Review." *Nutrients* 15, no. 23 (November 24, 2023), 4916. doi: 10.3390/nu15234916. PMID: 38068774; PMCID: PMC10708264.

Mehler, P. S., and A. E. Andersen. *Eating Disorders: A Guide to Medical Care and Complications.* Baltimore: Johns Hopkins University Press, 2010.

Mountjoy, M., K. E. Ackerman, D. M. Bailey, L. M. Burke, N. Constantini, A. C. Hackney, I. A. Heikura, A. Melin, A. M. Pensgaard, T. Stellingwerff, J. K. Sundgot-Borgen, M. K. Torstveit, A. U. Jacobsen, E. Verhagen, R. Budgett, L. Engebretsen, and U. Erdener. "2023 International Olympic Committee's (IOC) Consensus Statement on Relative Energy Deficiency in Sport (REDs)." *British Journal of Sports Medicine* 57, no. 17 (September 2023), 1073–97. doi: 10.1136/bjsports-2023-106994. Erratum in: *British Journal of Sports Medicine* 58, no. 3 (February 7, 2024), e4. doi: 10.1136/bjsports-2023-106994corr1. PMID: 37752011.

Mountjoy, M., J. Sundgot-Borgen, L. Burke, S. Carter, N. Constantini, C. Lebrun, N. Meyer, R. Sherman, K. Steffen, R. Budgett, and A. Ljungqvist. "The IOC Consensus Statement: Beyond the Female Athlete Triad—Relative Energy Deficiency in Sport (RED-S)." *British Journal of Sports Medicine* 48, no. 7 (April 2014), 491–97. doi: 10.1136/bjsports-2014-093502. PMID: 24620037.

Stellingwerff, T., I. A. Heikura, R. Meeusen, S. Bermon, S. Seiler, M. L. Mountjoy, and L. M. Burke. "Overtraining Syndrome (OTS) and Relative Energy Deficiency in Sport (RED-S): Shared Pathways, Symptoms and Complexities." *Sports Medicine* 51, no. 11 (November 2021), 2251–80. doi: 10.1007/s40279-021-01491-0. Epub 2021 Jun 28. PMID: 34181189.

7
SAMPLE MEAL PLANS AND SELECTED RECIPES

INTRODUCTION

The following sample meal plans are designed for a general guideline. They are not necessarily meant to be followed exactly, and definitely don't need to be followed on a long-term basis. They are simply a way to see what a normal day of eating might look like, with regular meals and a regular distribution of nutrients. Normal eating patterns like this help promote regular fueling, normal digestion, appropriate blood sugars, and adequate energy availability.

Since each person has unique nutrition needs, these meal plans will likely not meet yours. They are just here for some general guidance. Think of it as an example of what someone could eat in a day—because that is exactly what it is!

SAMPLE MEAL PLANS

DAY 1: 2,100-CALORIE MEAL PLAN

Food	Quantity	Calories (kcal)	Carbs (grams)	Protein (grams)	Fat (grams)
Breakfast					
Steel-cut oats	1.5 c	226	36	11	5
Blueberries	50 berries	40	8	0	0
2% milk	1 cup	125	12	9	5
Omelet	2 large	188	1	13	14
	Meal Totals:	579	57	33	24
Lunch					
Bread, whole-wheat	2 slices	153	22	8	2
Butter, without salt	1 pat	37	0	0	4
Baby carrots	2 medium	7	1	0	0
Cheese, cheddar	1 oz	115	0	7	10
Romaine lettuce	47g	8	1	1	0
Ranch dressing	1 tbsp	65	1	0	7
Canned tomato soup	1 cup	139	23	6	3
	Meal Totals:	524	48	22	26
Dinner					
White rice	1¼ cup	268	59	4	0
Grilled chicken	4 oz	249	0	27	19
Bell pepper strips	1 pepper, chopped	32	7	0	0
Cheese	¼ c shredded	114	1	5	9
	Meal Totals:	663	67	36	28
Snack					
Cheese, Colby	1 oz	112	1	7	9
Whole-wheat crackers	10 crackers	89	12	2	3
Grapes	10 grapes	55	10	1	0
Walnuts	10 walnuts	147	2	3	15
	Meal Totals:	403	25	13	27
	Plan Total:	2,169	197	104	105

DAY 2: 2,100-CALORIE MEAL PLAN

Food	Quantity	Calories (kcal)	Carbs (grams)	Protein (grams)	Fat (grams)
Breakfast					
Strawberries	1 cup, sliced	53	8	1	1
Greek yogurt, nonfat	1 container	100	6	17	1
Granola	1 oz	139	13	4	7
	Meal Totals:	292	27	22	9
Snack					
PowerBar®	1 bar	247	43	10	2
	Meal Totals:	247	43	10	2
Lunch					
Baby carrots	2 large	11	2	0	0
Grilled chicken breast	1 large fillet	242	0	49	5
Cucumber	21g	3	0	0	0
Romaine lettuce	94g	16	1	1	0
Italian dressing	2 tbsp	71	4	0	6
Tomato	68g	12	2	1	0
	Meal Totals:	355	9	51	11
Snack					
String cheese	1 piece	77	1	7	5
Dried apricot	1 oz	56	13	1	0
Pistachios	1 oz (49 kernels)	324	10	12	26
	Meal Totals:	457	24	20	31
Dinner					
Green beans, cooked	1 cup	44	6	2	0
Cheese, cheddar	½ cup, shredded	230	2	13	19
1% milk	½ cup	53	6	4	1
Whole-wheat pasta, cooked	1 large portion	358	63	14	4
	Meal Totals:	685	77	33	24
Snack					
Baby carrots	2 large	11	2	0	0
Cucumber	21g	2	0	0	0
Hummus	3 tbsp	75	4	4	4
Green pepper slices	46g	8	1	0	0
	Meal Totals:	96	7	5	4
	Plan Total:	2,132	187	141	81

DAY 3: 2,100-CALORIE MEAL PLAN

Food	Quantity	Calories (kcal)	Carbs (grams)	Protein (grams)	Fat (grams)
Breakfast					
Avocado	½ avocado	114	6	1	11
Multigrain bread	2 slices	138	19	7	2
Boiled egg	2 eggs	155	1	13	11
	Meal Totals:	407	26	21	24
Lunch					
Grilled chicken breast	5 oz	181	0	37	4
Grapes	10 grapes	74	17	1	0
Romaine lettuce	1 oz	4	0	0	0
Mushrooms	1 oz	8	1	1	0
Onions	garnish	2	0	0	0
Teriyaki sauce	1 tbsp	16	3	1	0
	Meal Totals:	285	21	40	4
Snack					
Peanut butter	2 tbsp	383	11	14	33
Rice cakes	2 cakes	70	14	2	1
	Meal Totals:	453	25	16	34
Dinner					
Green leaf lettuce	1 oz	6	1	1	0
Italian-style meatballs	3 pieces	160	3	8	12
Whole-wheat pasta, cooked	1½ cups	358	63	14	4
Vinaigrette	1 tbsp	72	0	0	8
Pasta sauce	½ cup	132	15	4	4
Tomato	5 slices	9	1	0	0
	Meal Totals:	737	83	27	28
Snack					
Low-fat chocolate milk		194	28	12	4
	Meal Totals:	194	28	12	4
	Plan Total:	2,076	183	116	94

DAY 1: 2,500-CALORIE MEAL PLAN

Food	Quantity	Calories (kcal)	Carbs (grams)	Protein (grams)	Fat (grams)
Breakfast					
Pancake mix	1 cup	437	74	26	4
Strawberries	5 strawberries	25	4	1	0
Lowfat Greek yogurt	1 container (7 oz)	146	8	20	4
	Meal Totals:	608	86	47	8
Snack					
Apple	1 apple	57	11	0	0
Peanut butter	2 tbsp	191	6	7	16
	Meal Totals:	248	17	7	16
Lunch					
Whole-wheat pita	1 pita	168	32	6	1
Cheddar cheese, shredded	½ cup	230	2	13	19
Green leaf lettuce	1 leaf	1	0	0	0
Orange	1 orange	45	9	1	0
Turkey slices	4 slices	60	1	10	1
	Meal Totals:	504	44	30	21
Snack					
Grapes	1 cup	113	26	1	0
	Meal Totals:	113	26	1	0
Dinner					
Meatless bacon bits	1 tbsp	33	1	2	2
Boiled broccoli	½ cup, chopped	27	3	2	0
Cheese, cheddar	1 oz	115	1	7	10
Grilled chicken breast	5 oz	181	0	37	4
Sour cream	4 tbsp	143	3	2	14
Sweet potato, cooked	1 medium sweet potato	235	45	5	0
	Meal Totals:	734	53	55	30
Snack					
Almonds	1 oz	164	3	6	14
1% milk	227 g	122	18	8	2
	Meal Totals:	286	21	14	16
	Plan Total:	2,493	247	154	91

7 / SAMPLE MEAL PLANS AND SELECTED RECIPES

DAY 2: 2,500-CALORIE MEAL PLAN

Food	Quantity	Calories (kcal)	Carbs (grams)	Protein (grams)	Fat (grams)
Breakfast					
Banana	1 banana	90	20	1	0
Quick oats	¾ cup	455	69	16	8
Walnuts	20 walnuts	262	3	6	26
	Meal Totals:	807	92	23	34
Snack					
Part-skim mozzarella	1 oz	72	1	7	5
Whole-wheat crackers	10	177	23	4	7
	Meal Totals:	249	24	11	12
Lunch					
Avocado	2 slices	34	2	0	3
Canned black beans	1 cup	218	23	15	1
Cheese, cheddar	½ oz	57	0	3	5
Long-grain cooked brown rice	2 cup	497	97	11	4
Salsa	2 tbsp	21	3	1	0
	Meal Totals:	827	125	30	13
Snack					
Baby carrots	10 medium	35	5	1	0
Hummus	2 tbsp	50	3	2	3
	Meal Totals:	85	8	3	3
Dinner					
Apples	1 apple	31	6	0	0
Brussels sprouts	½ cup	28	4	2	0
Grated Parmesan	1 tbsp	21	1	1	1
Grilled chicken breast	7 oz	181	0	37	4
Olive oil	1 tsp	37	0	0	4
	Meal Totals:	298	11	40	9
Snack					
Peanut butter	2 tbsp	191	6	7	16
Bagels	2 bagels	78	15	3	0
	Meal Totals:	269	21	10	16
	Plan Total:	2,535	281	117	87

DAY 3: 2,500-CALORIE MEAL PLAN

Food	Quantity	Calories (kcal)	Carbs (grams)	Protein (grams)	Fat (grams)
Breakfast					
Smoothie	1 smoothie	245	17	12	11
Muffins, oat bran	1 muffin	305	49	8	8
	Meal Totals:	550	66	20	19
Snack					
Boiled egg	2 eggs	205	2	17	14
	Meal Totals:	205	2	17	14
Lunch					
Grilled chicken	7 oz	181	0	37	4
Grapes	10 grapes	74	17	1	0
Romaine lettuce	1 oz	4	0	0	0
Mushrooms	1½ oz	8	1	1	0
Onions	garnish	2	0	0	0
Teriyaki sauce	1 tbsp	16	3	1	0
	Meal Totals:	285	21	39	4
Snack					
Peanut butter	2 tbsp	383	11	14	33
Rice cakes	2 cakes	70	14	2	1
	Meal Totals:	453	25	16	34
Dinner					
Green leaf lettuce	1 leaf	6	1	1	0
Frozen Italian-style meatballs	3	160	3	8	12
Whole-wheat pasta, cooked	1½ c	358	63	14	4
Vinaigrette	1 tbsp	72	0	0	8
Pasta sauce	½ cup	132	15	4	4
Tomato	2 oz	9	1	0	0
	Meal Totals:	737	83	27	28
Snack					
Whole-wheat crackers	12 crackers	239	33	6	8
Turkey jerky	1 package	64	4	12	0
	Meal Totals:	303	37	18	8
	Plan Total:	2,533	234	137	107

DAY 1: 3,000-CALORIE MEAL PLAN

Food	Quantity	Calories (kcal)	Carbs (grams)	Protein (grams)	Fat (grams)
Breakfast					
Whole-wheat bread	3 slices	230	33	12	3
Butter	1 tbsp	105	0	0	12
Scrambled eggs	4 large	364	4	24	27
Onions	garnish	2	0	0	0
Spinach	1 handful	0	0	0	0
Tomatoes	1 oz	6	1	0	0
	Meal Totals:	707	38	36	42
Snack					
Trail mix	½ cup	347	34	10	22
	Meal Totals:	347	34	10	22
Lunch					
Apple	1 apple	89	18	0	0
Whole-wheat bread	2 slices	153	22	8	2
Jam	1 tbsp	56	14	0	0
Peanut butter	2 tbsp	191	6	7	16
Plain, whole-milk Greek yogurt	1 container	121	5	11	6
	Meal Totals:	610	65	26	24
Snack					
Breakfast smoothie	1 smoothie	245	17	12	11
	Meal Totals:	245	17	12	11
Dinner					
Baby carrots	2 large	11	2	0	0
Minestrone	10 oz	226	32	10	3
Romaine lettuce	1 cup	8	1	1	0
Vinaigrette	1 tbsp	72	0	0	8
Sourdough bread	2 slices	231	42	0	3
	Meal Totals:	548	77	11	14
Snack					
Beverages, nutritional shake mix, high protein, powder	16 oz	470	25	64	13
	Meal Totals:	470	25	64	13
	Plan Total:	2,927	256	159	126

DAY 2: 3,000-CALORIE MEAL PLAN

Food	Quantity	Calories (kcal)	Carbs (grams)	Protein (grams)	Fat (grams)
Breakfast					
Apple	½ apple	31	6	0	0
Banana	½ banana	67	15	1	0
Quick oats	½ cup	148	24	6	3
Honey	1 tbsp	64	17	0	0
1% milk	½ cup	53	6	4	1
Walnuts	2 oz	392	4	9	39
Flaxseed	1 tbsp, ground	37	0	1	3
Ground cinnamon	½ tsp	3	0	0	0
	Meal Totals:	795	72	21	46
Snack					
Baby carrots	4 medium	14	2	0	0
Cucumber,	5 slices	7	1	0	0
Hummus	½ cup	204	10	10	12
Green pepper slices	5 slices	9	1	0	0
	Meal Totals:	234	14	10	12
Lunch					
Apple	1 apple	98	20	0	0
Wheat bagel	1 bagel	245	44	10	2
Cheddar cheese, shredded	½ cup	230	2	13	19
Romaine lettuce	1 leaf	1	0	0	0
Tomato	2 slices	6	1	0	0
Turkey slices	3 slices	45	1	7	1
	Meal Totals:	625	68	30	22
Snack					
Grapes	60 grapes	187	42	2	0
Almonds	1 oz	170	3	6	15
	Meal Totals:	357	45	8	15

(continued)

DAY 2: 3,000-CALORIE MEAL PLAN (*continued*)

Food	Quantity	Calories (kcal)	Carbs (grams)	Protein (grams)	Fat (grams)
Dinner					
Broiled beef tenderloin	7 oz	446	0	43	29
Boiled potatoes	1 potato	136	29	3	0
Zucchini	1 zucchini	27	4	2	1
	Meal Totals:	609	33	48	30
Snack					
2% cottage cheese	½ cup	279	17	36	8
Pineapple	1 cup, chunks	74	20	1	0
	Meal Totals:	353	37	37	8
	Plan Total:	2,793	269	154	133

DAY 3: 3,000-CALORIE MEAL PLAN

Food	Quantity	Calories (kcal)	Carbs (grams)	Protein (grams)	Fat (grams)
Breakfast					
Scrambled eggs	1 cup	273	4	28	16
Pork sausage	4 oz	379	2	16	34
Tortilla	1 tortilla	146	23	4	4
	Meal Totals:	798	29	48	54
Lunch					
Whole-wheat bread	4 slices	306	44	16	4
Butter	2 pats	74	0	0	8
Baby carrots	2 medium	7	1	0	0
Cheddar cheese (shredded)	½ cup	230	2	13	19
Romaine lettuce	1 oz	8	1	1	0
Ranch dressing	1 tbsp	65	1	0	7
Canned tomato soup	2 cups	277	47	12	6
	Meal Totals:	967	96	42	44
Dinner					
Salsa	4 tbsp	21	3	1	0
Quinoa, cooked	1 cup	222	34	8	4
Sautéed sweet red peppers	1 cup chopped	141	5	1	14
Sliced beef fajita strips	3 pieces	318	8	51	9
Black beans	1 cup	161	24	14	1
	Meal Totals:	863	74	75	28
Snack					
Cheese, Colby	1 oz	112	1	7	9
Whole-wheat crackers	10 crackers	89	12	2	3
Grapes	1 cup	55	10	1	0
Walnuts	50g	147	2	3	15
	Meal Totals:	403	25	13	27
	Plan Total:	3,031	224	178	153

RECIPES

EGG CUPS

12 eggs
½ c shredded cheddar cheese
4 tbsp bacon bits
2 sliced green onions

Combine all ingredients in a mixing bowl. Pour into greased muffin tins. Bake at 375 degrees for 10–15 minutes or until set up and no longer soft in the middle. Store in refrigerator. Microwave 1–2 at a time as desired for about 30–45 seconds. Makes 12 bites.

Nutrition information per bite:

- 100 calories
- 7 g fat
- 140 mg sodium
- 1 g carbohydrate
- 8 g protein

ENERGY BITES

1 c rolled oats
1 c shredded coconut
⅓ c sunflower seeds
½ c chocolate chips
½ c peanut butter
½ tsp vanilla
⅓ c honey

Combine all ingredients in medium mixing bowl. Scoop out a portion of about 2 tbsp, roll into a ball between your hands, and place on baking sheet. Repeat until the dough is gone. Place baking sheet in refrigerator for 15–30 minutes to chill the bites. Store in airtight container in the fridge. Makes 15 bites.

Nutrition information per bite:

- 190 calories
- 12 g fat
- 5 mg sodium
- 18 g carbohydrate
- 4 g protein

PROTEIN PANCAKES

- 1 egg
- 1 banana
- 2 scoops protein powder
- 2 tbsp flour
- 1 tsp baking powder
- ½ tsp vanilla
- ½ tsp cinnamon

Combine dry ingredients. Combine wet ingredients in separate bowl. Add wet to dry. Whisk together. Heat pan on stove on medium heat. Pour ½ cup of batter into pan. Let cook on one side until the batter forms bubbles and looks less shiny. Flip the pancake. Let cook 30–60 seconds longer or until cooked through.

Nutrition information for the whole recipe:

- 700 calories
- 10 g fat
- 760 mg sodium
- 104 g carbohydrate
- 51 g protein

BREAKFAST SMOOTHIE

- 1 handful washed spinach leaves
- ½ c frozen strawberries
- ¼ c frozen blackberries or blueberries
- ½ c Greek yogurt
- 1 oz chia seeds

Combine all ingredients in a blender. Blend until smooth. You may have to add 1 tbsp–¼ c water to make it a smoothie consistency, depending on the water content of your berries.

Nutrition information for entire recipe:

- 240 calories
- 11 g fat
- 105 mg sodium
- 31 g carbohydrate
- 12 g protein

ULTRALIGHT RECIPES FOR USE IN THE BACKCOUNTRY

LOADED BAKED POTATO SOUP

½ c instant potato flakes
¼ c whole milk powder
1 Tbsp bacon bits
½ Tbsp dried chives
¼ tsp garlic powder
⅛ tsp black pepper
2 × ¾ oz cheddar cheese sticks
2 Tbsp crispy fried onions

Home directions:

Put all ingredients except fried onions and cheese in a bag or container to be used in the backcountry.

Store the fried onions and cheese sticks in two separate bags or containers. The onions can be added to the soup mix but will lose their crispy texture when prepared.

Field directions:

1. Cut or tear the cheese sticks into small pieces and add them to the soup mix bag.
2. Add 10 oz (300 mL) boiling water to the bag or container.
3. Stir to mix well.
4. Put the bag or container in an insulated cozy to encourage total cheese melting.
5. Let stand for 5–10 minutes, allowing the cheese to melt and the potatoes to thicken to desired consistency.
6. Add the crispy fried onions, stir to mix well, and enjoy.

Nutrition information:

527 calories
25 g protein
41 g carbs
28 g fat

Recipe courtesy of backcountryfoodie.com. Used with permission.

BACON & EGG OATS

½ c rolled oats
2 Tbsp whole egg crystals
2 Tbsp Parmesan cheese
1 Tbsp bacon bits
1 Tbsp freeze-dried green onions
Salt and pepper to taste
2 Tbsp French-fried onions
1 Tbsp olive oil
10 oz water

Substitutions: Plant-based bacon bits may be used as a vegetarian option. Grated cashew cheese may be used as a dairy-free option.

Home directions:

Put all ingredients except oil in a bag or container for use in the backcountry. If you want the onions to stay crispy, place them in a separate bag.

Put olive oil in a leak-proof container. We recommend double-bagging the oil in the event of a leak.

Field directions:

1. Bring the water to a boil.
2. Put the dry ingredients in the pot. Reduce heat and simmer for 5 minutes.
3. Stir frequently to prevent the eggs from sinking to the bottom and burning.
4. Remove the pot from heat and add 1 Tbsp olive oil. Add the onions if you placed them in a separate bag.
5. Stir well and enjoy! The meal will continue to thicken if allowed to stand after removing from heat.

Nutrition information

470 calories
20 g protein
32 g carbs
31 g fat
626 mg sodium

Recipe courtesy of backcountryfoodie.com. Used with permission.

CHOCOLATE PEANUT BUTTER SHAKE

½ c whole milk powder
¼ c peanut powder
1 packet (1.26 oz) Carnation Instant Breakfast Essentials™ powder, chocolate

Home directions:

Put all ingredients in a bag or container for use in the backcountry.

Field directions:

1. Add 8 oz cold water to the bag or container. Add more or less water as needed to reach desired flavor.
2. Stir or shake vigorously to mix well.
3. Massage the bag with your fingers or use a utensil to break up any lumps. Enjoy!

Nutrition information

620 calories
39 g protein
63 g carbs
23 g fat
400 mg sodium

Recipe courtesy of backcountryfoodie.com. Used with permission.

DAYBREAK NUT BRAN

½ c raisin bran cereal
⅓ c whole milk powder
2 Tbsp sliced almonds
2 Tbsp chopped pecans

Note: non-dairy milk powder may replace whole milk powder for a vegan alternative.

Home directions:

Put all ingredients in a bag or container to be used in the backcountry.

Field directions:

Add 8 oz cold water. Stir well and enjoy!

Nutrition information:

496 calories
17 g protein
43 g carbs
30 g fat

Recipe courtesy of backcountryfoodie.com. Used with permission.

GARLIC HUMMUS

½ c dry hummus mix
1 tsp garlic powder
1 tsp dried parsley
Dash cayenne pepper
2 Tbsp olive oil

Home directions:

Put all ingredients in a bag or container to be used in the backcountry.

Put olive oil in separate leakproof container to be added when the meal is consumed. We recommend double-bagging the oil in the event of a leak.

Field directions:

1. Add 6 oz cold water or to desired consistency.
2. Stir to mix well until a smooth consistency is achieved.
3. Add olive oil.
4. Stir to mix well and enjoy!

Nutrition information:

571 calories
13 g protein
47 g carbs
39 g fat

Recipe courtesy of backcountryfoodie.com. Used with permission.

PORTABLE RICE BALLS

2 c uncooked rice (sticky rice like sushi or Calrose rice works best)
3 c water

Combine water and rice in a rice cooker; let cook according to the machine's directions. Alternately, cook on the stove in a pot by letting the water boil, adding the rice, and turning down the heat to low. Place lid on pot. Let the rice cook for 10–20 minutes or until the rice has absorbed the water and is no longer crunchy. Drain any excess water.

Shape the cooked rice into balls. Bake on a baking sheet lined with parchment paper at 350 degrees for 10–15 minutes.

Let cool, then wrap with plastic wrap or foil. Store in fridge. Take on hiking trips, skiing, bike rides, etc.

Tasty additions:

- Soy sauce
- Sesame seeds
- Chopped, pitted dates
- Chopped ham or Spam
- Shredded coconut
- Furikake seasoning
- Salt and pepper
- Peanut or almond butter
- Mini chocolate chips
- Substitute broth for water when cooking the rice
- Honey
- Mashed banana
- Raisins
- Spices (cinnamon, turmeric, nutmeg, seasoning salt, garlic, etc.)

Note: To follow best food safety practices for rice, consume these within 2 hours of taking them out of the fridge. You can also prep the rice before cooking it by soaking it in a solution of 300 ml of water plus 1 tbsp of 3 percent hydrogen peroxide for 5 minutes. Rinse the rice, then cook as directed. This reduces the risk of food poisoning from a bacteria called *bacillus cereus*.

Nutrition information for entire recipe made with no add-ins:

1430 calories
26 g protein
317 g carbs
2 g fat
4 mg sodium

DIY SPORTS DRINK

16 oz water
16 oz fruit juice of choice
¼ tsp salt

Combine. Enjoy.

Nutrition information:

223 calories
0 g protein
52 g carbs
1 g fat
575 mg sodium

DIY SQUEEZES

Think of these as a portable smoothie in a pouch. You can purchase reusable silicone pouches from many online retailers. Similar to commercially packaged applesauce pouches, these are portable food options that can relieve the taste fatigue of using store-bought gels.

The concept is to basically blend anything that sounds tasty to you, and pour it in the pouch. A funnel can come in handy for this step. Remember, always test your stomach tolerance during training. Don't try a new food on a race day or big trip where you may be stuck in the backcountry with gastrointestinal issues.

Be cautious with food safety. The pudding recipe needs to be consumed within 2 hours of taking it out of the fridge, due to the yogurt content. Recipes that contain mostly fruit and honey or syrup may last longer, especially if you are outdoors in cold weather.

The anatomy of a squeeze is simply a pureed fruit or vegetable, a honey or syrup, and a nut butter or spices as desired. You can invent your own combinations to suit your taste preferences. Rice gives it a more stable texture and adds carbohydrate content.

SWEET POTATO SQUEEZE

⅓ c cooked rice
2 tbsp cooked sweet potato
2 tbsp apple juice
1 tbsp honey
Dash cinnamon

Combine in a blender. Pour into the pouch. Enjoy!

Nutrition information:

165 calories
2 g protein
40 g carbs
0 g fat
13 mg sodium

CHOCOLATE PROTEIN PUDDING SQUEEZE

  1 c Greek yogurt
  ½ c protein powder (any flavor of your choice)

Combine. Add a small amount of milk as needed if the consistency is too thick. Pour into portable silicone pouches. Refrigerate. Consume within 2 hours of taking it out of the fridge.

STRAWBERRY SQUEEZE

  ⅓ c cooked rice
  5 strawberries
  ¼ banana or ¼ c applesauce
  1 tbsp honey
  2–3 tbsp water

Combine in a blender. Pour into the pouch. Enjoy!

Nutrition information:

  196 calories
  2 g protein
  48 g carbs
  3 mg sodium

DIY SPORTS GEL

This uses maltodextrin, which is a quickly digesting carbohydrate that is effective for fueling activities. Fructose is added as an additional carbohydrate. Since your gut can only absorb a finite amount of certain carbohydrate molecules at a time, using different carbohydrate molecules allows for better absorption and less gastrointestinal distress.

You can buy these from many online retailers. The beauty of these homemade gels is you can make up your own flavors, and they are much cheaper than store-bought gels. Using a kitchen scale to measure the ingredients is more accurate than measuring cups and spoons to get the proportions of ingredients correct.

HAYDEN'S GOO GEL

- 63 g maltodextrin
- 63 g fructose
- 2 g (1 tsp) sodium citrate
- 90 g juice or half juice, half water

Sift maltodextrin into a pourable vessel such as a large Pyrex. Add the rest of the ingredients and whisk with a fork until smooth. Pour mixture into a reusable pouch such as a Hydrapak 150 ml flask, which is equivalent to about 5 standard gel servings.

Nutrition total (150 ml): 527 kcal, 137 g carbs, 550 mg sodium
Nutrition per "gel" (25 ml): 105 kcal, 27 g carb, 110 mg sodium

Recipe credit: Hayden James, RDN, CSSD, CD, CDCES, www.satiatenutrition.com

Acknowledgments

Aaron Owens Mayhew, MS, RDN
Backcountry Foodie LLC
backcountryfoodie.com
Instagram: @backcountry_foodie
Facebook: @Backcountry Foodie

Morgan Arritola
Former Professional Endurance Athlete
2010 Olympian
Licensed Professional Counselor

Amity Warme, MS, RDN
Professional Rock Climber
Registered Dietitian
Amitywarme.com

Alyssa Leib, MS, RD
Peak to Peak Nutrition
www.peaktopeaknutrition.com
Instagram: @alyssaoutside_rd

Hayden James, RDN, CSSD, CD, CDCES
Satiate Nutrition
www.satiatenutrition.com
Instagram: @satiatenutrition

Index

acclimatization, 48–49
acetazolamide (Diomax), 48
acute injuries, 78
adaptive athletes, 72–75
adenosine triphosphate-phosphocreatine system (ATP-PC system), 6, 85
aerobic metabolism, 6
airplane travel, 75–77
alcohol, 12, 13, 80
algal oil, 59, 92
altitude considerations, 44–48, 51, 100
amino acids, 86–87, 94
amputees, 74–75
anaerobic glycolysis, 6
anorexia nervosa, 147–48
anthropometrics and climbing ability, 127–28
anxiety, 62
appetite, loss of, 44, 46, 48, 49–50
ARFID (avoidant restrictive food intake disorder), 150–51
Arritola, Morgan, 103
ATP-PC system (adenosine triphosphate-phosphocreatine system), 6, 85
avoidant restrictive food intake disorder (ARFID), 150–51

beet juice, 47
beta-alanine, 86–87
biking, 128–31
binge drinking, 12
binge eating, 37–38, 149–50
blood sodium, 133
blood sugar, 7–8, 62, 70
body image disturbances, 66
bone density, 66, 72, 74
bone injuries, 79
bonking, 7
Boone, Amelia, 147
brain health, 66, 85
brain injuries, athletes with, 74
Bratman, Steve, 152–53
bulimia nervosa, 148–49
Burke, Louise, 39

caffeine, 21, 76, 88–89
calcium, 58, 71, 79
calories, 30, 46, 52–53
See also energy needs
campground safety, 134–36
camping activities, 134–40
carbohydrates
   caffeine and, 89
   carb loading, 115–16
   complex carbs, 109
   female athletes' needs, 70
   intake recommendations, 8, 13, 27, 31–33
   mixing sources of, 32, 63, 117
   REDs and, 156
   role of, 5–8, 13
   simple carbs, 5–6, 20–21, 33, 38, 52, 64, 129
   in sports drinks, 20–21, 63–64
cerebral palsy, athletes with, 74
chronic injuries, 78
climbing
   anthropometrics and, 127–28

hydration and fueling during, 120–23, 126, 127
   tips from Amity Warme, 124–26
coffee and caffeine, 16, 21, 76, 88–89
cold weather, 51–53, 100–104
collagen, 79, 92–94, 95
concussions, 80
cortisol, 47
creatine, 59, 80, 85–86
cross-country skiers, 102–3

dehydration, 1, 17, 62, 63, 75
digestive issues
   diarrhea, 62, 63–64
   fiber and, 57
   supplements and, 86, 88, 89
   troubleshooting, 60–64, 117
Diomax (acetazolamide), 48
disordered calorie tracking, 30
disordered eating
   about, 145–47
   anorexia nervosa, 147–48
   avoidant restrictive food intake disorder, 150–51
   binge eating, 149–50
   bulimia nervosa, 148–49
   climbers and, 127
   healthy behaviors to combat, 160–62
   kids and, 66
   orthorexia, 152–54
   other specified feeding and eating disorders, 151–52

189

REDs and, 157
treatment for, 161
See also relative energy deficiency in sports (REDs)

electrolytes
  hydration and, 18, 46, 50, 62, 75, 106, 117
  in sports drinks, 20–21, 63–64
  wall climbing and, 126
Energy Availability Method, 28
energy needs
  about, 2–5
  calculating, 28–31
  campfire analogy, 5
  in cold climates, 52–53
  fluctuating during menstrual cycles, 70
  systems and substrates, 5–6
  See also food; fueling for special adventures; relative energy deficiency in sports (REDs)
equipment for camping, 136
estrogen, 70–71

fats
  food sources, 11, 13
  intake recommendations, 12, 13, 33–34
  role of, 5–6, 10–11, 13
  saturated *vs.* unsaturated, 11
female athletes
  amenorrhea, 157
  menstrual cycle phases, 64, 69–71
  osteoporosis, 157
  in perimenopause and menopause, 72
  pregnant athletes, 71–72
  triad patterns, 157
  See also disordered eating

fiber, 57, 64
fish oil, 59, 80, 91–92
fluids
  about, 16–17
  carrying, 22, 101, 128
  cool drinks, 50
  dehydration, 1, 17, 62, 63, 75
  overhydration, 18, 50, 62
  potable water, 136
  sweat rates, 18–20, 50–51, 62
  See also electrolytes; hydration for special adventures
food
  before, during, and after workouts, 38–39, 99
  carrying, 102, 117
  female athletes' needs, 70
  healthy *vs.* unhealthy relationships with, 160–62
  nutrition periodization, 39–40
  remembering to eat and drink, 123
  snacks, 76–77, 108–9, 110
  under-fueling, 66, 123, 126, 127
  vitamins and minerals in, 14–16
  See also fueling for special adventures; macronutrients; meal planning; menu samples
food/body/exercise relationships, 160–62
foodborne illness, 48
food poisoning, 62, 63–64, 77
food safety, 134–36, 185
fructose, 32, 33, 63
fruits and vegetables
  avoiding, 48, 63, 124

benefits of, 14–16, 23, 79, 90–91
as carbs, 8, 13, 107
in meal planning, 26–27, 55–56, 110
supplements and, 79, 90–91
vegan/vegetarian diets, 56–60, 94
fueling for special adventures
  biking, 128–31, 132–34
  camping, 136
  climbing, 99, 120–23, 124–25
  in cold weather, 52, 102–3
  at high altitudes, 44, 47
  hiking, 104–5, 106, 107–10
  in hot weather, 48–51, 66–67
  trail running, 113–19
  water sports, 132–34
  See also fluids; food

gastrointestinal issues. *See* digestive issues
glucose, 6, 7, 32, 33, 63
glycogen, 7, 49, 50, 51–52, 115, 134

Harris Benedict equation, 29
head injuries, 80
healing process, 77–80
heartburn, 61
high altitudes, 44–48, 51, 100
hiking trips
  challenges of, 104–5, 110
  common METs, 111
  fueling for, 106, 107–10
  hydrating for, 106–7
  sample meal plan, 110
  water purification systems, 107
hot weather, 48–51, 66–67
hunger cues, 115–17

hydration for special adventures
   biking, 128, 130–31
   camping, 136
   climbing, 120, 124–25
   in cold weather, 51, 53, 100–101
   at high altitudes, 44, 46–47
   hiking, 106–7
   in hot weather, 50–51
   trail running, 111–13
   water sports, 132, 133–34
   See also electrolytes; fluids
hyperosmolar solution, 62–63
hyponatremia, 18

intense workouts, 27, 31, 33
iron levels, 45, 57–58, 71

jet lag, 76
Jeukendrup, Asker, 39

kilocalories, 2
   See also energy needs
kilogram conversion, 8

lactic acid system, 6

macronutrients, 31–34
   See also alcohol; carbohydrates; fats; protein
maltodextrin, 187
masters nutrition, 67–68
Mayhew, Aaron Owens, 107, 109
meal planning
   calculating energy needs, 28–31
   for camping, 136–40
   carb loading, 116
   for climbing, 125–26
   consistency and timing of fueling, 5, 25–26, 36–39, 99
   easy meal ideas, 35, 56
   for hiking, 110
   macronutrients and, 31–34
   nutrition periodization and, 39–40
   plate method, 26–27, 31, 38
   See also food; menu samples; nutrition strategies; recipes
melatonin, 76
menopausal athletes, 72
menstrual cycle phases, 64, 69–71
menu samples
   for 2,100-calories, 166–68
   for 2,500-calories, 169–71
   for 3,000-calories, 172–75
   for biking, 130–31
   for hiking, 110
metabolic equivalents (METs), 29–31, 72–74, 100
   biking, 129
   climbing, 123
   hiking, 111
   specific sports, 104
   trail running, 119
   water sports, 133
metabolic rate, 51–52
micronutrients. *See* vitamins and minerals
Mifflin-St. Jeor equation, 28
moderate training days, 27, 31

National Eating Disorder Association, 153–54
National Institutes of Health (NIH), 13–16
nausea, 50, 61–63
NIH (National Institutes of Health), 13–16

nitrates, 90–91
nitric oxide, 47
nonbinary persons, 68–69
nutrient-dense food, 108–9
nutrition periodization, 39–40
nutrition strategies
   about, 1–2, 42–43
   for digestive issues, 60–64
   for extreme temperatures, 42, 48–51, 52–53
   goals, 99
   for high altitudes, 45–48
   for injury and surgery, 77–80
   masters nutrition, 67–68
   for para/adaptive athletes, 72–75
   planning, 42–43
   travel considerations, 75–77
   vegan/vegetarian concerns, 56–60
   for youth and adolescents, 64–67
   See also food; fueling for special adventures

older athletes, 67–68
omega-3 fatty acids, 59, 80, 91–92
orthorexia, 152–54
OSFED (other specified feeding and eating disorders), 151–52
osteoporosis, 157
other specified feeding and eating disorders (OSFED), 151–52
overeating, 37–38
overhydration, 18, 50, 62

para-athletes, 72–75
perimenopausal athletes, 72
plate method, 38
post-workout recovery, 5
potable water, 136

pound to kilogram conversion, 8
Predictive Equation Methods, 28–29
pregnant athletes, 71–72
progesterone, 70–71
protein
　for biking, 134
　for climbing, 121
　female athletes' needs, 70
　food sources, 9, 13
　intake recommendations, 10, 13, 26–27, 33–34
　role of, 9, 13
　in special situations, 79
　timing of consumption, 5
　in vegan/vegetarian diets, 60
protein powders, 94–95
puberty, 66

race day fueling plan, 119
recipes
　Bacon & Egg Oats, 179
　Breakfast Smoothie, 177
　Chocolate Peanut Butter Shake, 180
　Daybreak Nut Bran, 181
　DIY sports drink, 184
　DIY sports gel, 187
　DIY squeezes, 185–86
　Egg Cups, 176
　Energy Bites, 176
　Garlic Hummus, 182
　Loaded Baked Potato Soup, 178
　Portable Rice Balls, 183
　Protein Pancakes, 177
relative energy deficiency in sports (REDs)
　about, 154–57
　budget analogy, 154–55
　disordered eating and, 157
　high fiber meals and, 57
　menstrual cycle and, 71
　potential impact of, 145
RV life, 53–56

Schofield equation, 29
scurvy, 110
shelf-stable ingredients, 55
simple carbohydrates, 5–6, 33, 38, 52, 64, 129
sleep at high altitudes, 45
smart devices, 30
s'mores, 140
snow sports, 100–104
sodium, 18, 64, 117
　See also electrolytes
sodium bicarbonate, 87–88
spinal injuries, athletes with, 74
sports drinks, 20–21, 63–64, 184
　See also electrolytes
sprints, 6
stomach upset, 61
supplements
　about, 82–83, 90
　algal oil, 59
　beet juice, 90–91
　beta-alanine, 86–87
　collagen, 92–94
　creatine, 59, 85–86
　fish oil, 59, 80, 91–92
　kids not needing, 67
　protein powders, 94–95
　safety of, 83–84, 91, 92, 94
　in vegan/vegetarian diets, 58–59
　See also vitamins and minerals
sweat rate calculation, 18–20, 50–51, 62

taste fatigue, 114, 123, 131, 185

third-party testing of supplements, 83–84
time zone crossings, 76
trail mix, 139
trail running, 111–19
training days
　heavy, 27, 31, 33
　light, 27, 31
transgender persons, 68–69
travel nutrition, 75–77

ultrarunners, 114–15
under-fueling, 66, 123, 126, 127
urine color, 17, 18, 44, 47, 50, 53, 62, 120

van journeys, 53–56
vegan diets, 56–60, 94
vegetables. See fruits and vegetables
vegetarian diets, 56–60
vitamins and minerals
　about, 13–16
　B12, 58–59
　C, 45, 93, 110
　calcium, 58
　D, 58, 102
　iron, 45, 57–58
　sports drinks and, 21
　in vegan/vegetarian diets, 57–60
　zinc, 59
　See also supplements
vomiting, 61–63

water purification systems, 107
water sports, 131–34
weather extremes
　cold, 52, 102–3
　heat, 48–51, 66–67
wheelchair athletes, 72–74

young athletes, 66, 67

192　INDEX

About the Author

Marisa Michael, MSc, RDN, CSSD has been a registered dietitian since 2002. She holds a master's degree in sports nutrition, the International Olympic Committee's Diploma in Sports Nutrition, and is a Board Certified Specialist in Sports Dietetics. She owns a private practice in Portland, Oregon, where she does one-on-one consultations, workshops, and freelance writing. She also serves on the USA Climbing Medical Committee and has published peer-reviewed scientific literature. She is the author of *Nutrition for Climbers: Fuel for the Send.*

She grew up enjoying the outdoors and regularly enjoys paddleboarding, skiing, hiking, climbing, and triathlon. She bases her dietetic practice on evidence and science, marrying it with honoring the lived experience of her clients and their own food preferences and intuitive eating. She helps clients find ways to fuel their health and activities in a gentle way that makes sense to them. Her mission is to help people find better mental and physical health and performance through nutrition. You can find her online at realnutritionllc.com, nutritionforclimbers.com, or on Instagram @realnutritiondietitian.

FALCONGUIDES®

MAKE ADVENTURE YOUR STORY™

Since 1979, FalconGuides has been a trailblazer in defining outdoor exploration. Elevate your journey with contributions by top outdoor experts and enthusiasts as you immerse yourself in a world where adventure knows no bounds.

Our expansive collection spans the world of outdoor pursuits, from hiking and foraging guides to books on environmental preservation and rockhounding. Unleash your potential as we outfit your mind with unparalleled insights on destinations, routes, and the wonders that await your arrival.

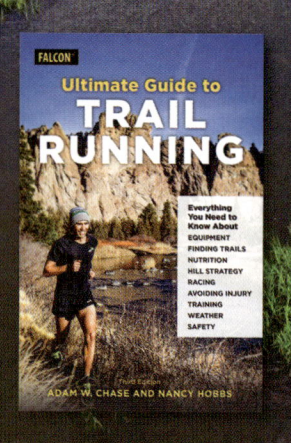

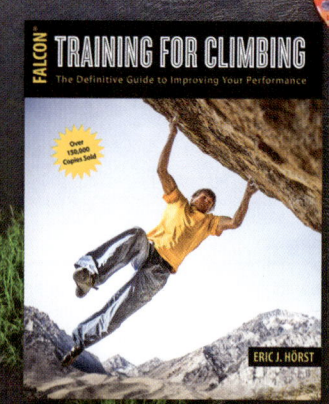

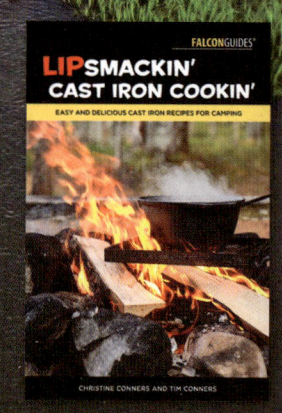

LET FALCON BE YOUR GUIDE

Available wherever books are sold.
Orders can also be placed at www.globepequot.com,
by phone from 8:00 a.m. to 5:00 p.m. EST at (800) 223-2336,
or by email at purchaseorders@simonandschuster.com.